What Is Z-Health?

The System That Eliminates Chronic Pain and Improves Athletic Performance

Jay Armstrong

Jay Armstrong
Copyright © 2017

ISBN: 099060392X
ISBN 13: 9780990603924

Foreword

"I'm old, tired, and I just don't want to learn anything new…"

This sentence is the punchline of a story that my dad told me many years ago. As we were driving to an appointment he started relaying a conversation he had the previous day with a friend of his regarding a new computer system that was being installed in their business.

His friend was complaining about all the changes and ended the conversation saying, "I'm old, tired, and I just don't want to learn anything new…" My dad said that was perhaps the saddest thing he had ever heard – especially considering that his friend was only 51 years old.

I tell you this story to emphasize the most important lesson I learned from my father – **relentless curiosity**. It was the trait I appreciated most about him and has served as a guiding principle in my life as well as in the development of Z-Health.

Z-Health, as a training system, is a reflection of this relentless curiosity. It is a system that continually evolves based on a burning desire to know more about the brain/body interface, as well as how to most efficiently fix it when it's broken and train it to be amazing.

Jay Armstrong, as a Z-Health Master Trainer, life-long high-level athlete and successful businessman is incredibly well qualified to write this book but not because of anything I just said about him. Rather, Jay is qualified because he is a perfect example of relentless curiosity and this book and its many lessons are the result.

I first met Jay several years ago as he began his journey through the Z-Health curriculum and I have watched him work his way through the many challenging paradigm shifts that he will share with you in the pages that follow.

One of the things that I have always loved about Jay is that he is what I call "old school" in his approach to things. He only talks about what he knows and he knows about things because he's done them – not just talked or read about them.

In this book, Jay does an amazing job of simplifying many of the complex neuroscience concepts of the Z-Health curriculum and personalizing them for you. Through his stories, experiences and great questions, Jay's book will take you on a deep dive into your own health and performance. He will challenge you to think differently and show you how to trust and train your body in ways that you have likely never experienced.

If you are simply looking for a book filled with Z-Health exercises you should probably put this one down and move on. If, however, you are looking for a book that can revolutionize your approach to rehabilitation and training you're in the right place.

If you have ever wondered what Z-Health is all about and if this "new" approach can benefit you, your family and your clients should dig into this book. Read it slowly, answer the questions and let it digest. Stay curious and if things in this book challenge your thinking then you know you're on the right track. More importantly, I know that if you apply what Jay has written you will feel the changes in your own brain and body beginning from the very first chapter.

When I am asked by students or other professionals how I designed the Z-Health curriculum I usually reply, "I try to only teach the classes that I wish I had been taught." I can say the same thing about Jay's book – he has written the book that he wishes he could have read about Z-Health from the beginning.

I think you will enjoy it tremendously. I know I did.

Dr. Eric Cobb -- Founder, Z-Health Performance

Preface

I have spent decades both working out on my own and training others. I wanted to be the best I could be, and I wanted to help others achieve their fitness and athletic goals. I now am painfully aware that I was making numerous mistakes throughout this period. I could have helped more people make faster progress. I could have avoided many injuries for myself and others. I believed much of what was written and said about health, diet, and fitness as though it was gospel. As it has been said many times, I wish I had known then what I know now.

I played football, basketball, baseball, tennis, and racquetball, and then I studied and competed in Tae Kwon Do. Over the past twenty years, I have had the great fortune to work with numerous exceptional athletes and trainers: Grand Master Y. D. Park, Master Kuk Chyung, Pavel Tsatsouline, Steve Maxwell, John DuCane, Gray Cook, Max Shank, and many more. Several years ago, I met Dr. Eric Cobb and began my study of Z-Health and brain-based training. This journey has led me to make a significant change to my paradigm about working out, exercising, and training. And this is what I hope to share with you.

Why didn't I improve faster? Why did many students develop injuries during their training programs? The old-school paradigm is that some people "had it" and others simply didn't. Those students who were gifted and talented picked up the sport and excelled. All they needed was desire. Those who were willing to work hard but had coordination issues or poor movement skills rarely if ever improved, and they were never able to play with the best.

Now I know that I could have done much more to help these athletes.

Here are few questions for you.

- Why are you exercising, working out, training, or dieting? Are you doing these things to "get into shape"? How will you actually know when you are "in shape"? Will that satisfy you? What will you do then?

- Are you exercising because your doctor or your peers told you that you needed to do this "for your health"? How do you know if what you are doing is improving your health or making you better? Is it possible that the exercise program you are following is actually making you worse or setting you up for an injury? Is that important to you?

- Do you want to change your physical appearance? What would it take to lose some body fat and to build some muscle? How much muscle do you want? How lean to you want to be? Do you want to be stronger, faster, or more flexible? How strong and flexible do you want to be? What are you willing to do to achieve this objective?

- Does exercising bring you joy? Do you have chronic pain? Can you perform any physical activity that you want whenever you want? Is mobility something that you want to possess?

These are difficult questions, and you may not want to face them. If so, then you might want to close this book and continue doing things exactly as you are doing them. This is what most people do. They do the same thing day after day and hope some change will magically occur. Of course, this doesn't happen. You will probably be unable to find any magic pill, potion, or lotion. If you continue to do the same thing day after day, then you cannot expect things to change.

> *All progress begins by telling the truth.*

Perhaps you want to continue on your current path because changing your paradigm is difficult. No, changing your paradigm is *really* difficult. The beliefs and values you hold — in fact, your concept of the world around you — has taken you a lifetime to formulate. However, changing your paradigm is what this book is all about.

If you are like me, then you know deep down inside that something about most current exercise and training systems in today's highly automated and fast-paced world just doesn't make sense. You "work out," but you don't get stronger or leaner. You don't know why you are working out, except that you know you should. You want to look better, but all the time you spend exercising doesn't really induce a change. You need to be "in shape" because your doctor and your friends say you must be. You are often sore, injured, and tired. And you don't really have the time or energy to devote to this project because you are busy taking care of your family and working to earn money.

How strong and lean do you want to be? Why? How much time can you devote to training? Is exercise something you dread? Or is your exercise program constantly being derailed because of your injuries and/or chronic pain?

I have good news! This book will help you change the lens through which you see yourself and your health. As a result, you will gain some clarity. You will have a much clearer vision for what you want to do when you "work out."

If, like me, you have exercised for your entire life, then you know that intense exercise can make you feel euphoric. In fact, exercise can be quite addicting. But does working out more and more make you better and better? Consider all the broken and unhealthy athletes who are engaged in CrossFit, long-distance running, or other endurance sports. Like all drugs, more is not necessarily better. What is the correct dosage? The answer is: it depends. This book will address the many factors that determine when and how you should push yourself to the next level and when you should back off.

> *Exercise is a drug. Too little won't do anything. Too much might be bad for you. Look for just the right amount to make you better.*

The brain is in charge of what we do and how we feel. One of the primary functions of the brain is to ensure our survival. In order to fulfill this assignment, the brain wants us to be smart, strong, and healthy, and it wants us to move well. This will allow us to find food, avoid danger, and create offspring.

We cannot do nothing all the time. Doing so will cause our brains and bodies to waste away. Conversely, there is a limit to what we can ask our bodies and minds to do based on our current health, strength, and abilities. So, we should find just the right amount of challenge. We must have sleep and recovery. We are looking for that sweet spot where we are challenged and we get better and not that excessive effort that breaks us.

You might be thinking that you need to push yourself so that you can expand your limits. That may be true. Feel free to put yourself through any extreme effort that you desire. The human body and mind are very resilient, and they can bounce back from virtually anything. But can you push yourself to your limits and beyond day after day? What price will you pay for that kind of behavior?

If the brain is in charge, then how can we determine what the brain wants us to do? The brain is a poor communicator. If you ask your brain, "Would doing five push-ups be good for me?" then the darn thing just sits there. Of course, we assume that if five push-ups are good for us, then fifty push-ups must be ten times better. Right? So, we ask the brain and again get that same lack of meaningful response.

Why is this? The brain is doing its job; however, we are poor listeners. The brain and body work together and give us feedback about many things, such as the need for sleep, food, water, and air. But we can get much more information and advice if we can develop the skill of being better listeners.

Unfortunately, we live in a world where we are taught that the growth of the mind is the responsibility of the school system. And we have the view that the repair and maintenance of the body is the responsibility of the medical system. We are free to do whatever we want, and when the body breaks, our doctor will do surgery or give us a drug to fix the problem. Part of this paradigm is that the brain and the body are separate entities. This is patently untrue, and somewhere deep inside, you know this is the case. Your brain cannot live independently—nor can your body. Your brain controls virtually all activities of the body. And without the body to protect and nourish it, the brain will die.

If you learn to listen more carefully, then the brain will tell you exactly what you need to do. The brain can communicate with you in the following ways:

- Weakness/strength
- Balance
- Fatigue/energy
- Peripheral vision
- Range of motion
- Endurance
- Mental acuity, focus, and creativity
- Reaction speed
- Pain

Now that we know how the brain talks to us, we simply need to implement a plan to listen to what it is telling us.

When the brain dislikes something we are doing, which one of these communication tools does it use? All of them. If you eat poorly one night, drink too much, and don't get enough sleep, then the result will be a brain/body system that performs poorly. Balance will be poor, fatigue will be high, endurance and strength will be compromised, and pain will be greater.

Here is the takeaway. When you are better, you are better. When you are worse, you are worse. When you are better, everything is better. When you are worse, everything is worse.

What is the purpose of exercise? Before answering that, we should define exercise. Exercise is what we do to prepare us for life's activities, maintain our health, and improve our athleticism. This is different from training. Training is working on a specific skill to support a specific sport, hobby, or goal. These are not mutually exclusive, but they are not the same thing.

The answer to this question is that there is only one purpose for exercise: to get better. If we get better a little bit each day, then eventually we will be really good. Can we do this by sitting in a car, sitting on a couch, or sitting at a computer workstation? It is highly unlikely.

What should we do in order to get better, healthier, faster, and stronger? What can we do to improve our range of motion and our balance? How can we learn to move without pain? Continue reading this book and prepare to be amazed at what we know about the human mind. This will hopefully begin to change the way you view yourself and the role of exercise in your life. As we move through these topics, I will recommend numerous excellent books. This is one of the greatest gifts that Dr. Eric Cobb and the Z-Health program gave me and that I am now sharing with you. You won't need to spend hundreds of hours looking for just the right book. Unless otherwise stated, each of these books is entertaining and nontechnical, but they help shed light on a pertinent and current subject. If the subject interests you, then I suggest you get the recommended book or the audio version to learn more than is presented here.

Contents

Introduction

Has anyone told you that you should check out Z-Health? Or perhaps you have actually met a Z-Health trainer and wondered, "What the heck is this Z-Health thing, and what can it do for me?" These are the questions that this book will help begin to answer. The Z-Health organization is headquartered in Tempe, Arizona, and is dedicated to providing cutting-edge education and training in the field of neuroscience and athletic skill enhancement. Z-Health is the very best system for relief of chronic pain. But it is also a system for improving athleticism. In fact, this is where Z-Health originally came from — improving performance.

Z-Health trainers very often obtain results with clients that seem magical. But there is absolutely no mystery, trickery, or sleight of hand involved. It is applied, cutting-edge neuroscience combined with practical physiological rehabilitation. Wouldn't it be great if I could move better and remain pain free into advanced age? I have two young boys, and I intend to run, jump, play, hike, and climb with them for many, many years to come. I am incredibly thankful for what the study of Z-Health has done for me and for thousands of others. My athletic abilities have improved, and my chronic pain has been virtually eliminated. I believe this is an incredible gift, and I want to share some of this system with you.

You are an amazing creature. Some humans can perform extraordinary feats of strength, mobility, balance, endurance, and reasoning. We are highly adaptable. This is, in fact, exactly how these extraordinary abilities are developed. Dedicated individuals apply stresses and challenges to the body and brain over and over, day after day, until the desired changes occur, and the person can "suddenly" ride a unicycle, hit a golf ball, or play piano. In other words, the exercises we do and our training and practice efforts cause adaptive changes.

But not all adaptation is positive. Your chronic pain and the type of exercise you are doing are almost always linked together. Your movement practice may make you better and more athletic, or it may be introducing unathletic compensations that will lead to injuries.

Proper exercise and training can improve an average person's performance or take a skilled athlete to world-class performance levels. But notice that the primary goal is to become a better athlete and a healthier individual. The goal is not to become better at exercise, although this might and probably will happen. Developing an increasingly high tolerance to exercise may in fact make us less healthy or make us less efficient athletes.

> *The purpose of your training is not to test your tolerance to exercise but to move better and to become more athletic.*

Yes, your exercise program can be breaking you! But the principles in this book have helped numerous athletes achieve new personal best efforts in just a few minutes. This seems too good to be true, doesn't it?

Isaac Asimov once said, "Any sufficiently advanced technology is indistinguishable from magic." Unexpected results very often look like magic, but they are not. When we integrate the numerous and disparate fields ranging from science and physical therapy to orthopedics and neuroscience, spectacular results become the norm. This is what Z-Health does. We are going to violate the sanctity of our medical system. Surgeons do not often approach a problem from a neurological perspective. Nor do orthopedic surgeons often consider vision as a possible contributing factor to joint pain. It is precisely because we will cross the boundaries of so many entrenched medical disciplines that what I will share with you will likely shake up your established paradigm.

What is a paradigm? A paradigm is a collection of all the thoughts and opinions from which we construct our worldview. A paradigm is the philosophical and theoretical framework on which we base our assumptions. A paradigm is a belief system or a mental program that has almost complete control over our behavior. A paradigm shift, where we move from our existing worldview to a new paradigm, usually occurs after a fundamental concept has been proven to be false or is no longer useful. Paradigm shifts are traumatic, upsetting, difficult, or painful. An example of a paradigm shift occurred when the world was determined not to be flat. Another was when we learned that the sun, and not the earth, was the center of the universe. Both of these paradigm shifts really shook up the established beliefs of people of the time.

We now know much more about how the brain functions, and we know that it is constantly changing. We have the ability to change who we are, how we think, and how we move throughout our entire lives. We now also know much more about pain. Just because your shoulder has hurt for five years doesn't mean that your shoulder is broken or that it must hurt tomorrow. This knowledge can upset your existing paradigm.

Paradigm shifts are extremely difficult and uncomfortable, and we resist them with all our being. Paradigm paralysis often prevents us from seeing and accepting any ideas or concepts that conflict with our existing, well-established, and comfortably entrenched paradigm. When it comes to technology, the event that changes a paradigm is usually called a *scientific revolution*. For example, the earth is *not* at the center of the universe. The Z-Health concepts and principles I am about to share with you, taken individually, are usually quite easy to accept. However, together, they form a new paradigm that will be difficult for most people to embrace without a small amount of discomfort.

As an example, one of the paradigm shifts I have made during my life concerns smoking. As a child, everyone around me smoked cigarettes: my parents, aunts, uncles, and all their friends. While my parents told me that smoking was bad for my health, it appeared that everyone smoked, and they all seemed to enjoy it. There were frequent television commercials showing how happy people were while they smoked. In those days, people were usually smoking in television shows and movies.

Our belief systems are strongly influenced by the experiences of our childhood years. And what those around me did was more influential than what they said. For many years, I thought smoking cigarettes was a cool thing to do. Almost all my friends smoked cigarettes. Eventually, though, I was able to replace my childhood belief with a new one: "Smoking makes you smell like a dirty, old rug (or worse), and it is extremely bad for your health." Changing my paradigm was made more difficult by the fact that, in many cases, I chose to stop associating with some people because I didn't want to be put into a position where I had to smell and breathe someone else's smoke.

Another paradigm shift I made involved flexibility. I played high school football and was active in many other athletic activities. However, none of these required a significant level of flexibility; it was not emphasized, and we never did any real work on this skill. We were supposed to be strong and fast. Stretching was for sissies, dancers, or golfers (or so I thought). As a kid, I was fascinated with martial artists such as Bruce Lee. I assumed that they were born with the "flexible" gene. When I attended my first Tae Kwon Do class with Master Park, he led the class in warm-up exercises. At the end of the warm-up, I was in for a treat. He told us to sit on the floor and to separate our legs far apart. I could get them almost ninety degrees apart; however, to stay in this position, I needed to put my hands behind myself on the floor to hold me up. Then he told us to exhale and to put our chest on the floor between our legs in front of us. I started laughing. I couldn't sit in this position let alone bend forward! As I watched Master Park demonstrate, it seemed his body was made of rubber, and his legs were sticking out from the sides of his body. I thought it was very funny. Orientals were clearly much more flexible than American athletes. Weren't they?

I continued to attend Tae Kwon Do classes, working very hard in every class. I also practiced all the techniques at home, including the stretching drills. Very slowly, my range of motion and strength improved. Eventually, I was able to put my hands on the ground in front of me. Then my elbows made it. My feet were getting farther apart. Then my chest was on the ground. Had I become Asian? No. We get better at the things we practice. Our bodies adapt in response to the stresses applied. I had to change my paradigm from "It is impossible to perform these feats of flexibility" to "Anyone, given enough time and effort, can transform his or her body to achieve miraculous results." Changing my belief system did not happen easily or quickly; however, we can change our view if we want to badly enough.

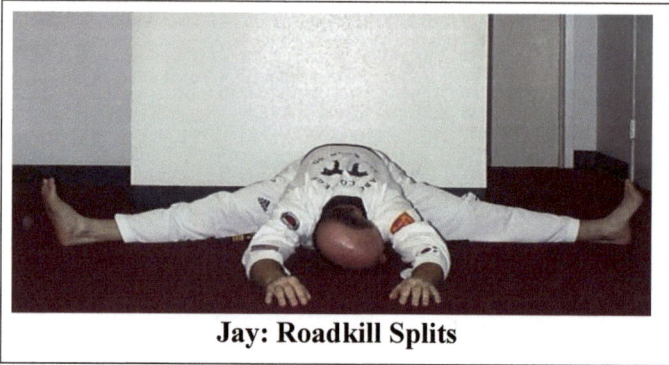
Jay: Roadkill Splits

A wide range of beliefs helps to form our concept of the world around us. This book is about many simple concepts that work together to form a cohesive picture. You will likely agree quite readily with most of these concepts, or at least they will not be off the charts in terms of being a possibility. However, taken together, they will challenge your current idea of what is important when it comes to exercise, health, chronic pain, and what you are capable of doing.

Let's see if you agree with these simple concepts that we are going to explore.

1. You want to get better. That's why you are reading this book: you are interested in changing your paradigm.

2. The brain and body are one system. The body supports the brain. A healthy body will better support and encourage proper functioning of the brain.

3. The brain controls the movements of the body and what we do with all our waking hours.

4. We are not a collection of body parts. The system is integrated, and everything works together. Each part has an effect on many other parts.

5. The brain is in charge. It processes the sensory input from the body, and based on that information, it decides what we will do next.

6. The purpose of the brain is to ensure our survival. To achieve this goal, the brain wants us to be healthy and athletic. This will help us avoid danger, find food, and create offspring.

7. The brain learns through a process we call *neural chunking*. For example, sentences are comprised of words, which are comprised of letters. First we learn the letters. Then we learn words. Then reading is possible and requires less effort. Once reading is mastered, we don't consciously think about the letters.

8. Emotion plays a role in the way new neural chunks are formed. If something is important or fun, then we can create a new neural chunk faster. The way to get rid of an old, bad, or inefficient chunk is to replace it with a new, good, or more efficient chunk.

9. The brain is constantly processing sensory inputs and interpreting that data. It is from this data that the brain forms a concept of the body and of the world around us.

10. The brain, outside of our conscious awareness, processes most of our sensory input. We would be overwhelmed if we had to pay attention to all visual, vestibular, and peripheral input.

11. Since the brain is primarily concerned with survival, it is constantly on the lookout for threats. All stress is a potential threat. Stress causes the brain/body system to work harder and to use more energy. Stress takes some of the brain's focus away

from other things like creativity, concentration, and quality movement.

12. The brain/body system is constantly adapting. New neural connections are being created, new memories are being formed, and the body is growing new skin, muscle, and bone.

13. We are all athletes, and everything is a skill. We can practice and get better at any skill. This means we can get better.

14. The brain contains maps of our body and the world around us. We can remap the brain with deliberate practice. The brain is plastic or malleable. Therefore, we can change how our brain functions.

15. Tissue and bone respond to stress. Bodybuilders create large muscles by lifting heavy weights. Our bodies can also create new bone structures as a result of the stresses they experience.

16. The high-tech, computer-centric American lifestyle causes numerous adverse physical adaptations: rounded shoulders, collapsed rib cages, shortened hip flexors, and compromised eyesight. In addition, supportive and heeled shoes cause adverse changes from the "normal" or optimal foot and ankle function.

17. You can build the body you want. Look at the bodies that power lifters, gymnasts, swimmers, and marathon runners have. Their bodies have adapted to the activities in which they are involved. You can also create changes in your body.

18. If you do what makes you a little bit better — every day — then you will eventually get much better. Conversely, if you are getting a little worse each

day, then eventually you will arrive in a very bad place.

19. Pain exists in the brain. It is a construct that occurs as the result of sensory input processed through experience. A paper cut can be excruciating. You might be cut and bleeding and not even know that it happened. Pain is an action signal. It is one of the ways that the brain communicates with you.

20. The brain tells you when you are hungry or thirsty or when you need to go to the bathroom. These are nonverbal communications. We can learn to listen to the instructions of the brain. (This is what potty training is.) If you listen to the brain/body system by performing self-assessment, then you can find out what the brain wants you to do so that you can get better.

21. We must focus on creating higher quality movement patterns. This will cause our brains, muscles, fascia, and bone to adapt to our new, more efficient movement skills. In short, we will build a better body.

22. Complex movements are comprised of smaller movements. Break movements and other complex tasks into their smaller components, get better at the components, and then reassemble the smaller components into the complex task.

23. We must constantly look for weaknesses or compromised movements. Then, if we can put aside our pride, we can work to reduce these weaknesses and to eliminate the compromised movements. Unfortunately, most of us want to work on those things at which we are already good at. It is humbling to address our areas of deficiency.

24. All movements have multiple components: range of motion, speed, and load. To truly own a movement skill, we must be able to perform it in a variety of postural positions, be able to execute it at various speeds, and be able to execute that movement skill with a variety of loads.

25. Sensory input plays a large role in developing and performing quality movement patterns. Properly functioning vestibular (or inner ear) and visual systems will reduce stress and help give the proper input that is essential for quality movement.

26. The responsibility is yours alone. Doctors, personal trainers, and coaches can help you with your journey, but ultimately, your ability to move well and to be healthy is up to you. You must have quality, focused practice in order to develop improved movement skills.

These concepts are not complex. Yet very few people incorporate them into their belief systems. As a result, they cannot act on them. However, the very reason that most people move poorly and have chronic pain is a direct result of not acting on one or more of these concepts.

We will look at these concepts in greater detail in the following chapters. As you can see, these concepts incorporate a wide variety of subjects. Throughout this book, I will introduce you to some exceptional resources that will expand on these topics should you be enthusiastic enough to want to delve more deeply into them. New ways of looking at and understanding the things we already know can often lead us to a slight shift in the way we think and can eventually guide us to a radically new paradigm.

Chapter 1: Adaptation

The human organism is incredibly adaptive. We can live at high altitudes, at sea level, and for a while, even in outer space or under water. We can build communities of igloos on the Arctic Circle, live in grass huts near the ocean, or raise our families in multifloored buildings in polluted cities. We can eat virtually anything: vegetables, meat, fish, eggs, seaweed, grain, chocolate shakes, and French fries. We can learn to sing and to acquire the ability to speak one or more languages. We can even learn to type, text, Tweet, and use the Internet. We can adapt to just about anything.

Examples of adaptation can be seen in the differences among world-class athletes. Speed skaters have large quads, while swimmers have uniquely well-developed shoulder musculatures. Or compare different types of runners. Milers are generally quite thin, while sprinters look more like bodybuilders. Our bodies change in response to the stimulus they receive. And this adaptation applies to much more than just our muscles. Everything in our body is constantly changing. We are rebuilding bone. This is necessary so that our bones can become stronger and so that they can repair themselves in case of a fracture. Our hair is growing. We generate new skin and blood cells every minute of every day. Our brains are forming the neural connections to support new skills and to build new memories. The entire body/mind system is constantly engaged in a process of regeneration and of restructuring itself to meet the current demands of its specific environment and doing what is necessary for us to survive in it. Fortunately, we can make good use of this ability to adapt. All we need to do is figure out how we want to adapt, make a plan to cause this adaptation, and then implement the plan. You can become the exceptional athlete you were meant to be.

> *You are constantly adapting—whether you want to or not.*

Wolff's Law and Davis's Law

Let's take a look at how this adaptive process works. In the nineteenth century, the German anatomist Julius Wolff observed that stress applied to bones causes changes to their structure. This is something most of us have already heard. It is recommended that women exercise with weights so that they will develop denser bones and help prevent osteoporosis. If you are a martial artist and you like to break boards or bricks on a regular basis, then your bones will also become denser in response to this practice (or abuse). Another vivid example of this adaptive process is dental braces. Wires are placed in the mouth and gently pull your teeth this way and that. As pressure is applied to a tooth, the bone dissolves on one side of the tooth and regrows on the other side. As you can see, even your bone structure is changeable. If you have a hunched back or flat feet, then the underlying bone structure has likely changed adversely over a period of many years. It did not suddenly appear one day.

This ongoing adaptation to applied force is one of the big problems facing astronauts. Bone loss can occur at a rate of up to 1.5 percent per month. We must apply force to our bone structures in order to maintain their strength. This is an excellent example of how we are constantly adapting whether we want to or not.

There is a corollary to Wolff's law, Davis's law, named after Henry Davis, which says basically the same thing about soft tissue. Muscles and tendons will become stronger if stressed and will become weaker if not used. In addition, muscles will become shorter if they are never elongated. We see examples of this type of adaptation in bodybuilders and power lifters who can pack on unbelievable amounts of muscle as a result of their constant exposure to the stresses of lifting and moving heavy weights. Similarly, dancers and contortionists can develop incredible flexibility and ranges of motion through their seemingly tortuous stretching practices. And, unfortunately, patients lying in a bed for an extended period undergo adverse changes to their muscles, becoming weaker and less flexible.

Now that we know our bones and soft tissues can adapt to externally applied stresses, what does this mean to us? The first thing it means is that this adaptation is going on all the time whether or not we want it to happen—all day, every day. If we are not applying stresses to our muscles and bones, then they will become weaker. Similarly, if we are constantly applying a stress, any stress, to our bodies, then we will see some adaptation. Unfortunately, not all adaptation is good. Imagine, for example, that you tied a leather strap to a five-pound weight, made a loop in the strap, put your arm through the loop, bent your elbow, and carried this weight around all day, every day. You would get pretty good at carrying this weight around, but your elbow might not straighten as well after many years of this practice. Although this may seem like a far-fetched example, there are many women who are walking around carrying their purses in exactly this manner—on the same arm every day. Could this behavior cause an adverse adaptive change? Yes, it could.

I once had an employee complain to me that her knee had begun to hurt, and she felt she needed to consult a doctor. For many years, I had observed that she spent much of the day, every day, sitting with one leg folded under her. Amazingly, the leg she was sitting on each day is where her knee pain was. I pointed this out to her. She stopped sitting on her leg, and miraculously, her knee pain began to subside.

As another example, if you spend eight hours each day with your shoulders forward and your chest collapsed, as you do when working at a computer, then you will get pretty good at this position. This position could also cause unwanted changes to your body.

Your bones, muscles, and other tissues are adapting all day, every day. The movements you choose to do each day (or the lack of movement you do each day) greatly affect this adaptive process. Much of what you do each day is done without conscious thought, but you are adapting anyway.

> *The body you have is the body you have earned through the way you move.*

The Modern Lifestyle

Technology has made our lives much easier. We can do research and order new toys without getting up from our desk. We constantly send texts and Tweets, write e-mails, and post new updates on Facebook. Our cars are so advanced that we don't need to turn our heads to back up and park. Our computers do our research for us so that we don't need to go to the library, pick up a book, and read. We can open a document on our screen, search for the information we want, and make the font as big as we need so that we can see it clearly. We can listen to most books in audio format. We have fast food and cushy shoes. Thus, we can gain all the weight we want, and there will be no shock from the impact of our feet on the pavement. Of course, we will park very, very close to the door of the store so that we don't need to walk very far. We have air-conditioning so we won't sweat, heaters so we won't be cold, and toilets that are very far from the ground so that we don't need to squat down too much.

Our modern, coddling lifestyle does not require a lot of physical effort, and as a result, we have developed bodies that are virtually incapable of hard work. This is a direct result of the maxim "you will get better at the things you practice." If you practice sitting, then you will actually adapt and become better and more efficient at this activity. You will develop the bone structures, ligaments, tendons, and muscles to support this activity. You will become a sitting machine! And you will develop habitual movement patterns based on the fact that most of your work and movement skills are performed while seated.

An ideal standing posture, the one we need to use when we are walking efficiently, positions the weight of the head over the shoulders. The shoulders are over the hips, the hips are over the knees, the knees are over the ankles, and the ankles are over the heels. In other words, we are properly aligned vertically to take maximum advantage of our skeletal structure. While standing, we have just the right amount of tension in the front of our body to balance the tension in the back of our body. This keeps us erect. We do not want any extra tension because this would be a waste of energy. If we are moving well—and this is what we are designed to do—then we are athletic, we are efficient, and our posture is erect and well aligned.

The Most Important Exercise

Movement is very important for our health and well-being, yet our modern lifestyle has done nearly everything possible so that we don't really need to move much at all. We have an incredible movement deficit. The end result is that now we have a dilemma. We need to find the time in our busy lives to exercise because we don't get quality movement challenges in our regular work activities. Daily lives used to be filled with lifting, working, painting, digging, washing, and so on. Humans are designed to work and move all day, every day. As a substitute for this lost behavior, we now hope to stay strong, mobile, and fit by exercising for a few hours each week. This is a real challenge. It is a battle that we are generally losing. We simply cannot get enough quality movement practice in such a short period of time. The amount of time spent moving is simply insufficient to undo all that other time spent in inactivity.

Certainly, we need to do some kind of exercise, and hopefully this physical activity will cause our bodies to undergo positive adaptation. We are in a hurry, so we need to find out how to maximize the time and effort of our movement practice. Don't we?

Let's think this through. You (or your trainer) might believe that the most important exercise we can do is the push-up or maybe the squat, right? Let's take the push-up as an example. If you did one push-up every day, then your body would undergo some kind of physiological adaptation. More significant changes would occur if you did one hundred push-ups every day. The more work you do, the more change you will no doubt see. Although you don't push up 100 percent of your body's weight during a push-up, for the sake of the following example, let's use simple math: if you weigh 150 pounds and do one hundred push-ups every day, then that is 150 pounds times one hundred reps, or fifteen thousand pounds of work. That's a pretty significant load, isn't it?

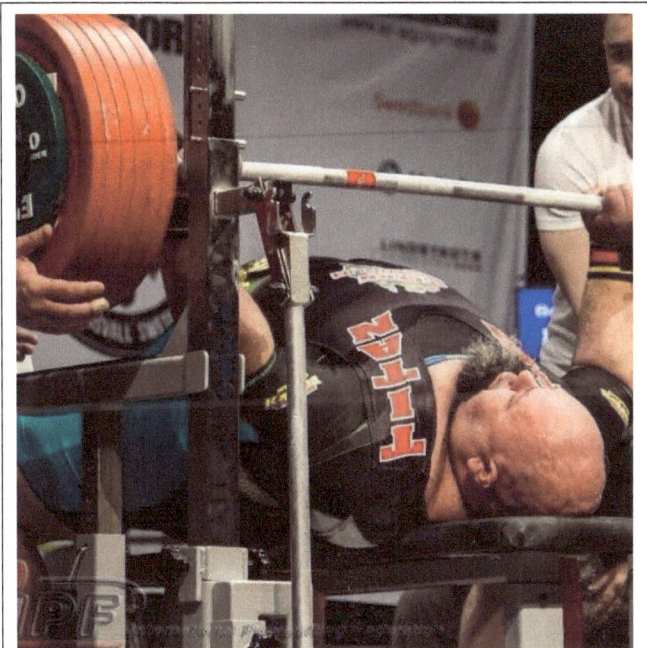

Nathan Baxter – Powerlifting Champion
Preparing for a Heavy Bench Press

What we intuitively understand from this mental process is that a greater load, increased intensity, higher repetitions, or a higher frequency in our exercise program will step up the adaptive process. Every physical activity you do causes your body to adapt in some way. However, the things we do most often or that involve the greatest loads will affect us more.

Let's assume that you occasionally go to the gym and work out and that you occasionally engage in some sports activity or play. Which exercise or activity is causing the greatest adaptive effect on your body? For ultra-runners, who can run one hundred miles or more at a time, it may be running. For long-distance cyclists, it may be riding a bicycle. But, for most people, including individuals who are exercising quite a bit, the answer is walking. I am not

18

talking about going for long walks with your friends but rather regular walking that happens all day, every day, like going to and from the refrigerator. Let's see why this is true.

According to the National Health Services of UK, the average person takes "between 3,000 and 4,000 steps per day."[1] Active people may take significantly more, on the order of ten thousand steps per day. If you own a Fitbit device, then ten thousand steps is the number they recommend you take daily. But four thousand steps per day is a common number even for sedentary individuals. How much weight or force are we talking about during each of these steps? The average person creates a force of two to three times his or her body weight during each footfall.[2] Using a sample bodyweight of 150 pounds, the math would look like this:

$$4,000 \text{ steps} \times 150 \text{ lbs.} \times 2 = 1.2 \text{ million pounds of force each day!}$$

Compare fifteen thousand pounds from the one hundred push-ups with more than a million pounds of force from even a moderate level of walking. This is almost one hundred times as much force being applied to your bones, ligaments, tendons, and muscles. And this is happening *every* day! These forces originate in the foot, but they travel up the leg, through the hip, and into the spine. And they don't stop there. These forces affect your neck, shoulders, knees, elbows, and virtually everything else in your body. The takeaway here is that how we walk can and does

---

[1] "The 10,000 Steps Challenge," National Health Services, Accessed February 24, 2017, http://www.nhs.uk/Livewell/loseweight/Pages/10000stepschallenge.aspx.
[2] "Biomechanics of Walking (Gait)," footEducation, Edited July 16, 2015, http://www.footeducation.com/foot-and-ankle-basics/biomechanics-of-foot-and-ankle/biomechanics-of-walking-gait/.

cause significant changes in our bodies' structures. These changes can be making us better or worse. They can make us more efficient athletes, or they can cause adverse adaptive changes. Could the way you walk cause you to experience shoulder pain or neck pain? Yes, it could. Could improving the way you walk make you a more efficient athlete and cause the brain to reward you with better balance and increased range of motion? Absolutely.

> *Walking is probably the most significant exercise you do to cause changes to your body.*

Chronic pain is a creation of the brain, and it is an action signal that tells you to do something differently. If your gate is poor, then the brain can create a pain experience to let you know that you are moving inefficiently. We will explore the brain and chronic pain much more later.

The Seated Position

Contrast the desired quality posture of a standing position with the everyday seated position. When you are seated at a desk and working on a computer, or when you are driving a car, your upper back (or thoracic spine) is rounded forward. This spinal flexion causes your shoulders to move forward and your upper arms (or the humerus bones) to rotate internally. A symptom of this internal shoulder rotation is that your elbows will move outward. This will make it easier to put your arms on the armrest of your chair.

Notice that when your thoracic spine is rounded forward and your shoulders are internally rotated, your head will move in front of your shoulders. This head-forward position is also encouraged by the fact that we instinctively want to get closer to our work. Of course, while you are seated, you are also bent at the hips. In other words, the hips are in flexion. For most people, when the hips are in flexion, the legs tend to externally rotate so that the knees move apart.

The miraculous human adaptive process is ongoing. We are adapting all day, every day. Let's do some more high-powered mathematics. Assume that you go to the gym four times per week for an hour each time. That's four hours of adaptation time. How much time are you spending seated at a computer, texting, or driving a car? Let's be conservative and say four hours of computer work and two hours of driving *every* day. That would be four hours of gym time each week compared with forty-two hours of sitting time *every* week. You are getting ten times the amount of practice at sitting as you are at whatever your exercise is. And, more than likely, you are sitting many more hours than this.

Here is the adaptation that occurs as a result of this large amount of time spent in the seated position. The head moves forward and becomes quite comfortable with this position. This increases the curvature of the neck (or cervical spine). The upper back, or thoracic spine, becomes stuck in a flexed or forward curved position. This interferes with our ability to breathe efficiently. The shoulders develop a preference for remaining in front of the chest with the arms internally rotated. This reduces our ability to move our arms overhead. The hip flexors, which are constantly flexed while in the seated position, no longer want to release to allow you to stand erect. This causes the pelvis to tip forward, spilling the belly and the contents of the guts outward. The legs that spend so much time externally rotated can remain that way as you walk. This external rotation causes the ankles to fall to the inside of the heel. When the ankles move inside the heels, our arches collapse, and we have flat feet.

This doesn't paint a very pretty picture, does it? What should you do? Should you stop sitting? Obviously, we cannot avoid sitting, and you don't need to. Everything that we do causes our body to undergo adaptive changes. And now that you know what all that time spent in the seated position is doing to you, you can incorporate some serious counteractive measures so that when you stand up and walk, you will be able to do so with the athletic efficiency you were meant to have. When you sit, be good at sitting. When you stand and walk, do this with proper and efficient posture. Until you recognize that this is a problem, you certainly cannot fix it, can you?

Vision

There is yet another unfortunate thing that happens from all that time spent sitting at a computer. What are you doing with your eyes during all this computer time? They are focused at "monitor" distance, somewhere between far away and up close. Also, your eyes are neither moving from side to side nor up and down. And what do you think your athletic eyes are designed to do? They should support athletic movement. This means they should be able to rapidly change focal length from near to far distances, scan the visual field for movement or dangers, and track objects as they approach us. When we don't move our eyes day after day and we don't change focal distance, we begin to lose those abilities. In other words, we are getting worse.

Thousands of years ago, humans walked around, searched for food and companionship, and avoided dangers. During all these activities, their eyes were moving left and right, changing focal distances, watching for movement, and absorbing information about the world around them. There are six muscles that control the movement of each of our eyes so that we can move them up, down, left, and right. These muscles are subject to the same laws as all the muscles in your body. You can strengthen them with daily use or appropriate exercise, but they will become weaker with nonuse.

Our hunter-gatherer forefathers mostly looked at objects in the distance while walking around, or they focused on objects near to them when they were working with their hands. Now, in the modern age, we spend countless hours with our gazed fixed on a computer screen that is neither near nor far but rather at monitor distance, with our eye-focusing muscle somewhere between completely relaxed and strongly contracted. The distance at which our eyes are focused doesn't change for hours at a stretch. What do you think is the result of these many hours of practice? We are getting better at focusing at monitor distance at the expense of our ability to rapidly change focal length from near to far and back again.

The primary function of the brain is to ensure your survival, and your visual skills are very important for this. The ability to scan the world around us and rapidly detect movement is an essential early warning system. In addition, the ability to see something in the distance and to change our focus as the object approaches is critical in order for us to avoid being struck by falling rocks, stung by bees, or impaled by flying spears. Flying spears may be over the top, but balls can be thrown at us, and cars are always trying to crash into us.

The point is that if your visual skills are compromised, then you will once again run the risk of making the brain unhappy. You have reduced the brain's ability to protect you from danger. Is it possible that the brain will try to "tell" you that you should do something to maintain or improve your vision skills? Yes, it is. And one of the ways that the brain communicates with us is via chronic pain. Can your gradually declining visual skills cause you to experience neck, shoulder, or some other pain? Yes, they can. Could working on your vision enhance your athleticism, make you move better, and improve your balance? Absolutely.

Shoes

The bone structures of your feet and ankles are very similar to those of your hands and wrists. We have the capability to use our feet in much the same way as we use our hands, and with practice, this can be achieved. Google "girl with no arms," and you will find a couple of videos on YouTube that show what can be done with your feet. These videos show women, born without arms, driving a car, typing, washing dishes, changing diapers, and putting on makeup.[3] The dexterity they have developed with their feet is simply amazing. This is one of the things that made Houdini such a great escape artist. He constantly worked on the dexterity of his feet and toes, and with them, he was able to tie and untie knots. People would tie up his hands, thinking he couldn't escape, and he would simply untie the knots with his feet! We are all born with the bone and muscle structures in our feet that would allow us to do these same things. We simply have not had enough motivation to develop those skills.

Now imagine what would happen if you took two pieces of leather, shaped them roughly into cones, stuck each hand into one, and snugly tied a string around each. And pretend that you did this every morning when you woke up and kept your hands like this all day, every day. What kind of adaptive changes do you think would occur to your hands? Nothing good. Your hands would lose their dexterity. Eventually, you would lose mobility in your wrists, and all fingers and would start losing their accurate sense of touch. Every day, you would be learning that you

---

[3] "Woman with No Arms—No Excuses," YouTube, Published June 27, 2014, https://www.youtube.com/watch?v=49hkD6dmX8k.

do not need to move your hands or feel anything with them. This is in essence what most people do with their feet. They stuff them into shoes and lace them up tightly. Most shoes are not shaped like feet but are in fact quite pointy. Unfortunately, your feet are not pointed and therefore must adapt to this strangely shaped piece of leather.

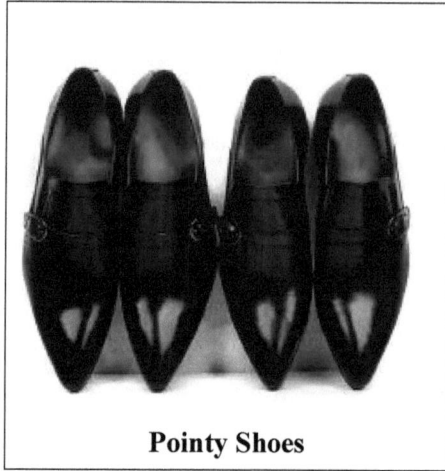

Pointy Shoes

In addition, most shoes have heels that range from a half inch to several inches. This includes men's shoes as well as ladies' shoes. Shoes with heels cause our toes to be below our heels. This places our ankles into a position called *plantar flexion*, with our foot pointing downward. The opposite position, with our toes pulled toward our shins, is called *dorsiflexion*. Both plantar flexion and dorsiflexion are required for normal ankle mobility. Spending all your waking hours in plantar flexion will cause physiological adaptation to the bone structures of your feet and ankles. This can lead to a loss of dorsiflexion. We must have adequate dorsiflexion if we want to possess efficient athletic movement skills such as the ability to squat.

Another strange thing that happens when we put a heel on our shoe is that our heel strikes the ground prematurely.

When this happens, it sends a significant shock up the leg and into the spine. Often, your feet, knees, or hips will begin to ache from this constant banging. What did the shoe industry do about this? Did they reduce the height of the heel? Of course not! They decided that the real problem was inadequate cushioning, so they made the heel bigger and even more cushy. This makes us hit the ground harder with our heel, but now it feels good to do so. Now we have a new and improved method of walking that allows us to slam our heels into the ground over and over, maintain our foot in plantar flexion, and begin the ongoing adaptive process to this rather unathletic gate pattern.

In addition, in an effort to ensure that no one ever twists an ankle, the shoe designers have made sure that we have adequate support on the sides of the ankle and heel. This is good, right? We all have weak ankles, and we might hurt ourselves. We can protect our ankles by adding lateral support, and the shoe companies are doing us a favor by providing it. Unfortunately, supporting your ankles or any other body part with an external device simply means that you don't need to do the job yourself. This will inevitably lead to additional weakening of the area you are trying to protect. Wearing high-top shoes and putting braces on both wrists, both elbows, and both knees will make you much weaker and put you at increased risk of injury in the long run.

Modern shoes put our ankles into plantar flexion, squish our toes together, and immobilize our heels and ankles. The foot and ankle are supposed to be mobile to absorb the forces of every step while we walk, but our feet are no longer mobile. Imagine trying to hike or run in ski boots. If you are unfamiliar with this piece of equipment, it is as rigid as a cast. The impact you feel when walking in ski boots is quite annoying.

Every day we spend in our tightly cinched up shoes causes our feet to adapt—to possess less and less sensitivity and mobility. Since our feet and ankles are not mobile, we are less athletic, and there is more hammering on the knees, hips, spine, and so forth. Is it possible that the chronic pain in your knee, shoulder, or neck is a signal from the brain that you should do something about the lack of mobility in your feet and ankles? Yes, it is possible. Could regaining proper sensory input from your feet and improving the shock-absorbing and supportive quality of your feet help you move better and have better endurance? Absolutely.

> *Rigid, supportive shoes cause reduced ankle and foot mobility, making us less athletic.*

Now, you might think that we need these cushy and supportive shoes in order to protect us when we are running. *Born to Run* is an excellent and entertaining book by Christopher McDougall.[4] In this story of the Tarahumara Mexican Indians, McDougall introduces us to the concept of barefoot running. And I am not talking about running around the block. Not even close! This tribe of Indians loves to run. They eventually become convinced to come to America and to join in some ultra-marathon events, races of more than one hundred miles. They might have worn some thin-soled sandals, but none of them wore Nikes or Adidas support shoes with air-cushioned soles.

---

[4] Christopher McDougall, *Born to Run: A Hidden Tribe, Superathletes, and the Greatest Race the World Has Never Seen* (New York, Vintage Books, 2009).

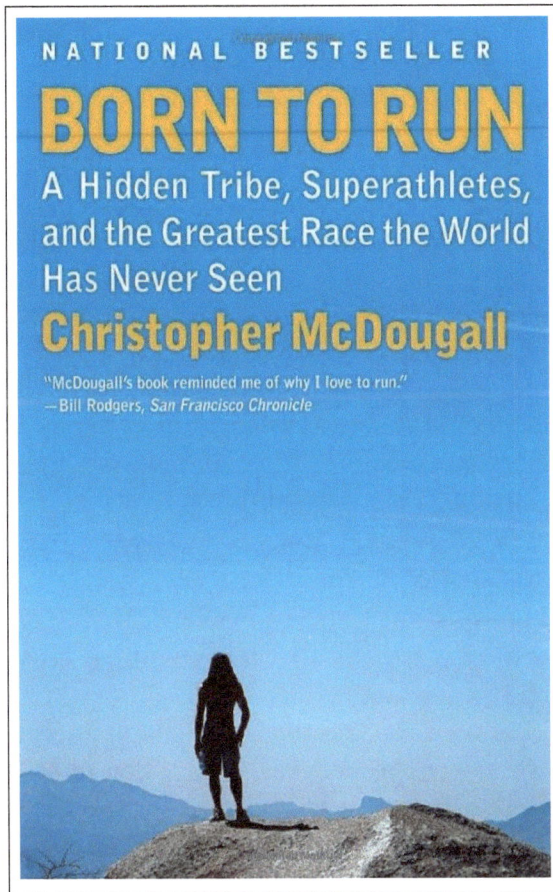

If our movement quality is good, then our feet are well designed to support our walking and running efforts. And strengthening our feet by spending more time barefooted or with minimal support from our footwear will help us develop our best possible movement quality. We will receive improved input from our feet and be better able to develop efficient, low-impact skills.

Movement Skills

The manner in which we move causes adaptation throughout the body. Because the brain controls our movements, the brain is also adapting as a result of our movements. That's right. The way we move causes changes in our brains. Our muscles, bones, tendons, ligaments, and even our brains are undergoing minute changes throughout the day as a result of what we do. The quality and frequency of our movement directly affects the brain and causes it to adapt. The brain is constantly processing sensory input from our body. The more we move in complicated ways, the wider the variety of sensory information that the brain must process. From these inputs, the brain constructs a view of our bodies, how we move, and the world around us. The loads we apply to our bones and muscles, following Wolfe's law and Davis's law, encourage their adaptation. The sensory inputs from our body cause our brain structures to adapt.

If we have weak muscles, malformed feet, poor vision, and fragile or twisted bones, then we are unlikely to move well. Therefore, we want to develop strong, functional bones and muscles to support efficient athletic movement. But the brain is also one of the structures of our physical being, and as such, it is also constantly adapting. Let's look at how our brain changes in response to our movement practice or lack thereof.

We have the ability to learn new words and to form new memories. These activities cause physiological changes to the structure of the brain. There is also an ongoing, adaptive process occurring in the brain as a result of your movement and from the associated sensory input. New neural connections are always being developed, discarded, or strengthened. If you don't perform movements such as playing a piano or hitting a golf ball, then your skill at these movements will decline. Similarly, regular quality practice can improve movement skills. Quality practice is the key phrase here. Randomly banging your hands on the keys of a piano will not improve your piano playing. The practice must be performed in a way that actually makes you better if that is your goal. And remember, your goal is pain-free exceptional athleticism. This goal simply cannot be achieved without regular practice at movement skills. Which movement patterns or skills should we be practicing? Only the ones that we want to remain good at. There is an old adage that goes like this: "Which teeth should you brush?" The answer: "Only the ones you want to keep."

Skill Development

How do we move? We don't actually know. We don't think about it. We just do it. If we had to analyze or think about which muscle should contract, how strongly it should contract, and exactly when this should happen, then we would not be able to move at all!

The way we move works something like this. First, we visualize, imagine, or feel what the movement will be like. In other words, we predict that the movement will occur. This is one of the reasons why watching someone else perform a movement helps us to do it. We have "mirror" neurons that help us use others' performance to visualize ourselves performing the movement.

Second, we perform the movement. During this process, we may use our cognitive abilities to think about or focus on one aspect of the movement we are doing. We are also processing the sensory input from our arms and legs and our visual and vestibular systems while we are executing the movement.

Third, we compare the movement we actually performed with the movement we had visualized. We evaluate how closely the outcome matches the desired result. This may or may not happen on a cognitive level, but it is happening.

These parts need not necessarily occur sequentially. If you are walking, running, or riding a bicycle, then you have an ongoing movement pattern with continuous evaluation of how well you are performing the movement.

We execute a complex program in the brain each time we move. This process causes thousands of neurons to fire in a sequence specific to that movement. As your neurons fire over and over again, they become faster and more efficient at that specific process. There are physiological changes that occur that cause the neurons to grow new dendrites, the long, thin connections at the end of each neuron, and to lay down insulation (or myelin) on the outside of the neurons. These physiological changes are persistent and allow you to get better at that particular movement skill over time.

This adaptation is more significant when you perform the movement frequently. In addition, this adaptation is affected by your emotions. If this activity is important to you, either because it makes you happy or because it is essential for your survival, then these physiological changes will occur more readily. Your emotion, focus, and interest act as catalysts to speed up the adaptive process.

In a similar manner, movements or skills that we do not use often or that are not important will also cause a physiological adaptation. The insulation (or myelin) will eventually be discarded. The brain, assuming that other skills, movements, and activities are more important, will work to create those new, efficient neural connections and allow the others to waste away. The brain is adapting just like the rest of the body, and it is subject to the same use-it-or-lose-it rules.

One of the purposes of the brain is to support movement. The brain controls all our movements, and it is constantly adapting. Therefore, it is essential that we do what is required to cause the brain to adapt in a way that will support the desired quality movement skills.

Bone and Tissue Remodeling

We now come back to Wolff's law and Davis's law and how they apply to the way you move. You are constantly building a new body, one that supports the movements you are doing every day.

If you spend a lot of time in front of a computer monitor, then you probably do this with your head positioned in front of your shoulders and chest. When you operate in this position for hours upon hours, the physiological adaptation is significant. The muscles, tendons, and fascia that work to support your head in this forward position begin to change so that it requires less effort for you to do this. The vertebrae in your neck also begin to change in response to the time spent in this position. Remember that the material in your bones is also being swapped out all the time. The shape of your cervical vertebrae will change over time based on the load applied to them, and you will develop stronger ligaments to help hold your head in this forward position.

Just as you may experience adverse adaptive changes from the head-forward, monitor-gazing position of your head and neck, your feet and ankles can become more or less able to support efficient athletic movement. Your habitual movement patterns and the associated stresses that are placed on the tissues and bones of your feet and ankles will cause the body to change the shape of these bones and to lay down new material on the nearby fascia, tendons, and ligaments.

Let's take a look at the anatomy of the ankle. Many people think of their ankles as the two bumps above each of the heels. The inside bump is called the *medial malleolus* and the outside bump is called the *lateral malleolus*. These malleoli are at the ends of the tibia and fibula, the two bones of the lower leg. We all know that the bone at the very bottom, where our bodies make contact with the earth, is the heel. But between the heel and the malleoli is another bone, the talus. The ankle is actually where the three bones, the tibia, the fibula, and the talus, meet. This ankle joint is meant to be strong and mobile. We should be able to move our ankles up and down and side to side through a wide range of motion.

A great amount of force is entering our body through our feet, and this will cause significant adaptive changes to the bone structure of our ankle. If our feet are externally rotated, our arches are collapsed, and our ankles are falling medially on every step during gait, then our bodies' structures will change to support this new movement pattern. Over time, we will get better at this movement, and we will develop the ideal body to allow us to move this way. As a result of this adaptation, however, we may not be able to move our ankles as they were originally intended. We might, as a result, not be the exceptional athletes we once were, and we might develop knee pain or hip pain from our ankles' movement dysfunction.

Our daily posture, the things that we do, and the ways that we move are causing us to change and to develop a new body. This body can be better and more athletically efficient. Or your body can be adapting in an unhealthy way to support repetitive, unathletic daily movements.

> *Your body is always adapting to exactly what it is doing.*

Your brain is aware of all this on a subconscious level, and your brain wants you to be an efficient athlete, capable of surviving and reproducing in this hostile world. Aware of adverse physiological changes, could your brain send you a signal to tell you to do something differently? Could your brain cause your knee to hurt so that you will perform some corrective exercises on your ankle or your neck? Yes, it could. Conversely, could working to regain normal function of your neck and ankles make you a stronger, more mobile, pain-free athlete? Absolutely.

Why We Have Joints

There are more than two hundred bones in the human body and more than two hundred articulating joints that connect those bones. What is the purpose of each of those joints? The answer is *movement*. When movement of a joint between two bones is no longer necessary, the bones begin to fuse together. A functioning, articulating joint requires maintenance and energy to keep it working properly. The body wants to minimize such energy expenditures. If you aren't going to use a joint, then you will be better served by its elimination and the creation of new bone to replace it. And if you aren't going to move a joint, then you must *want* it to stay in a fixed position. This is what a bone does. It is fixed and rigid. The system tries to help you out by getting rid of the joint and replacing it with a bone.

Having said all that, how many of your joints are supposed to move? *All* of them. And how do we keep a joint functioning? By moving it. Joints are different from muscles in that there is little blood flow bringing nutrients to the site and removing waste products. Joints have a liquid called *synovial fluid* in the joint capsule. Since the heart is not pumping this synovial fluid into and out of the joint, what encourages the flow of fluids necessary for maintenance? Movement! Your bodily movements lubricate the joint and act as the pumping mechanism for the lymphatic system. The lymphatic system is similar to the system of veins that courses through your body, but it is used to remove waste products, transport white blood cells, and recirculate plasma. A healthy lymphatic system requires you to use all the muscles in your body, and this means you must move.

Let's talk about how joints are supposed to move. There are different types of joints. The hip is a ball and socket type of joint, while the knee is a hinge type of joint. However, each joint has a range of motion that could be considered normal for a fully functional joint. For example, the elbow joint should be able to fully straighten (or extend), and it should be able to bend (or flex) to an angle greater than ninety degrees. Joint function obeys the use-it-or-lose-it rule. What we can infer from this discussion is that each of our joints should regularly be moved. And they should be moved through their full range of motion. The exact motion will be different for different types of joints and will vary from person to person. If we don't regularly move a specific joint through one part of its range of motion, then we run the risk of adverse adaptation and the possibility that that range of motion may no longer be available to us when we want it.

The muscles that cross a joint are responsible for the movement of that joint. And strength is an essential part of our athletic ability. For example, we should not only be able to bend our leg at the knee joint and then to straighten that knee joint but also be able to climb a flight of stairs while carrying a bag of groceries. This not only requires a certain amount of strength from the muscles but also applies a load to the joint structure. Therefore, another aspect of a joint's well-functioning behavior is to handle a variety of loads. This is a function of both the muscles that cross the joint and the health and proper operation of the joint itself. The brain receives a lot of sensory input from our joints, and if a joint is not healthy, then the brain can reduce the available strength of the associated muscles in order to protect that joint. In order to maintain the proper functioning of a joint, we must move the joint with a wide variety of loads applied. This not only will keep the joint working but also will help strengthen the associated muscles and connective tissues.

Finally, there is the matter of speed. You might be able to slowly rotate your head to the left and to the right, but if someone behind you yells, "Look out!" then you will try to look that way very quickly. If a joint will not move slowly, rapidly, and at all speeds in between, then the joint is not as useful as it could be. Perhaps you can move all your joints through a full range of motion at slow speed, but running, jumping, kicking, and throwing all involve the use of many joints, and some of them are moving rapidly.

To maintain the proper function of your joints, you must move all of them on a regular basis. All joints must be moved in a way that will take them through all their ranges of motion. In the case of highly mobile joints, such as the shoulder, there may be an incredibly high number of possible movement patterns. The arm can be moved in front of the body, across the body, overhead, and more while in either internal or external rotation. In addition to challenging the joints with a full range of motion, the joints and associated muscles must be able to cope with a variety of loads. This can be considered strength training or weight training. Perhaps a better way of viewing this training is that we are learning to move with a variety of loads: some heavy and some light. For example, a deadlift is basically standing up while holding on to a barbell.

Sometimes you might want to kick a soccer ball or throw a baseball. You could want to hit a tennis ball or a golf ball. Or you might need to chase your kid or run away from a bad guy. All of these are fast skills. Pouring water from a big bucket into many small bottles is a slow movement skill. We need to maintain all our joints, and to do these things, we must constantly challenge them by moving them through a full range of motion with a variety of loads at speeds ranging from slow to fast. This will ensure that we maintain or regain our exceptional athletic movement abilities.

> *Joints must be moved through all ranges of motion at a variety of speeds and with a variety of loads.*

The brain is aware of how all your joints are functioning, and it wants you be an exceptional athlete so that you can find food and avoid danger. Is it possible that your brain could send you a signal, such as reduced energy levels or compromised balance, to tell you to rehabilitate your compromised joint function? Yes, it could. Could you enhance your athletic performance, coordination, and endurance by improving the way each of your joints moves? Absolutely.

> *Each joint in our bodies must be moved on a regular basis in order to maintain proper function of that joint.*

Neural Connections

Our central nervous system is composed of cells called *neurons*. These neurons fire or transmit an electrical current when they are active. When a neuron fires, it can either encourage an adjacent neuron to fire or work to inhibit its ability to fire. This is the underlying process for memory, experiences, feelings, thoughts, and most functions of the central nervous system.

Many neurons fire in a complex and coordinated sequence for each movement we perform. The more accurately timed the sequence is and the more repeatable the firing of the desired neurons is, the better our skill at a particular movement will be. This is the essence of skill development. The rule is that deep, quality practice will make us better at our skills. All the activities we perform with our brain are subject to this rule.

> *Everyone is an athlete. Everything is a skill.*

In Daniel Coyle's excellent book *The Talent Code*, you will learn much about the coating on the outside of our neural pathways.[5] This white coating is called *myelin*, and it is much like the insulation on the outside of electrical wires. It is composed mostly of cholesterol. (All cholesterol is not bad for you.) Myelin helps prevent leakage of electrical current and ensures that the path of the current is accurate and distinct. Myelin also helps increase the speed of transmission. This means we are able to think and react more quickly. When we have practiced a movement or skill for thousands of hours or many years, the body lays down more myelin on the pathway associated with this movement. This is another reason why master musicians or exceptional athletes make their arts look so effortless. It does require less effort for them. They react more quickly, their movement sequences are more highly coordinated, and the amount of energy required for all this is less. This is what myelin does. This is what quality, deep practice does.

---

[5] Daniel Coyle, *The Talent Code: Greatness Isn't Born. It's Grown. Here's How* (New York: Bantam Books, 2009).

THE

TALENT

CODE

UNLOCKING THE SECRET OF SKILL

IN SPORTS, ART, MUSIC, MATH,

AND JUST ABOUT ANYTHING

DANIEL COYLE

author of the *New York Times* bestseller *Lance Armstrong's War*

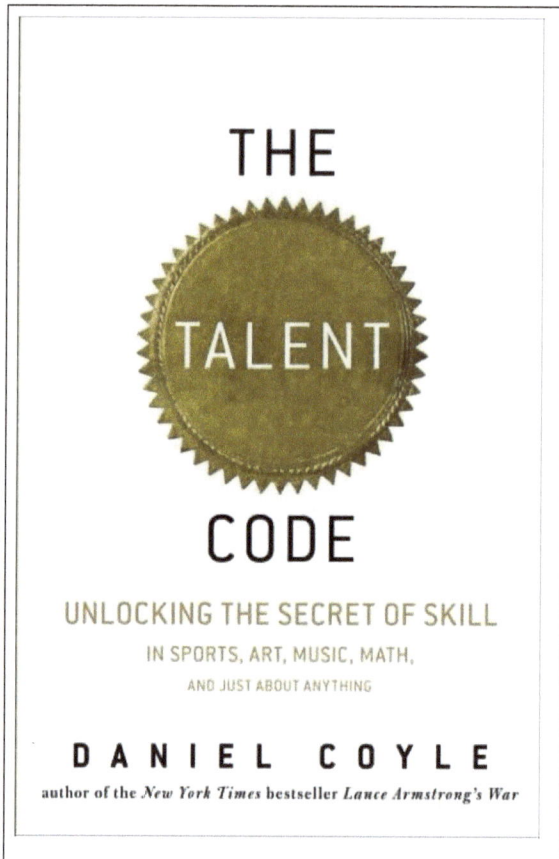

As you practice your movement skills, you are undergoing a physical transformation in the brain and throughout your nervous system. Neurons grow new dendrites, the tiny filaments on the ends of the nerve cells, and myelin forms around the neural circuits. In essence, through deep, deliberate practice, you are becoming a more efficient athlete, artist, or scientist. What happens when you stop practicing? The neural circuitry quality begins to decline. The body doesn't want to spend the energy to maintain something you are not going to use. When you stop practicing or performing your skill, the myelin coating on the nerve pathways will become thinner, transmission speeds will slow down, and the neural circuit will become less efficient. You will become a little worse each day at that activity.

This is not always a bad thing. We are infinitely adaptable. We can acquire skills for nearly anything we want. And when we don't need something, we can discard it. Many years ago, scientists and engineers performed calculations using a device called a *slide rule*. Using a slide rule required both an understanding of how to do the calculations using this tool and some physical skills in order to move the slide and the marker piece back and forth. Once the handheld calculator was readily available, the slide rule was obsolete. The calculator is more accurate, faster, and simpler. Engineers allowed those slide-rule skills to waste away, since they were no longer necessary.

But some skills slip away without our conscious awareness. Suppose that each day we lost a little more of our quality movement in our feet, ankles, eyes, and shoulders. We wouldn't even notice this until we suddenly discover we cannot squat, catch a ball, or raise our arms overhead. We will do ourselves a great service if we periodically do inventory of all our movement skills and ensure that we are still exceptional athletes. Skills can only be maintained through use and practice.

Takeaway

You are constantly adapting whether or not you want to, and due to our modern lifestyle, much of that adaptation is not good. Now, instead of moving all day, working at our job, lifting, crawling, twisting, walking, and so on, we must set aside a special time when we can do these things, a special time for "exercise." (Sounds like a four-letter word, doesn't it?) And when we find time in our busy lives for some exercise, what exactly should we do with this time to make the most of it? Surely, we want to get into shape. But I am not sure what that means to you. One focus of your exercise program might be to elevate your heart rate, and the heart is certainly a muscle. However, if you have poor movement quality and you apply a load to your movements, or you perform high repetitions of your poor movements, then you will not only elevate your heart rate but also more deeply ingrain those poor movement patterns and possibly put yourself at risk of injury. The purpose of any exercise program must be to get better. For nearly everyone in today's society, this means a significant portion of their "exercise" time should be spent on reversing the adverse adaptive changes that are occurring every day.

Our physical adaptation is not limited to muscles and bones. The brain is also constantly adapting, as is the rest of the nervous system. New myelin is being laid onto those circuits that we fire more frequently. We are either becoming better at a skill or our talent is declining.

A large part of our nervous system is designed to accept, transmit, and process sensory information, such as touch, pressure, temperature, and so on. If we don't move and thereby receive the necessary sensory stimulus, then this portion of our nervous system will begin to decline. With disuse, the ability to sense with our peripheral nerves will decline, and the ability of the brain to process that information will degrade as well.

Paradigm Shift

I played football through grade school and through my sophomore year in high school. Eventually, all the other players were *much* bigger than me, and I wisely decided I needed to find something else to amuse myself.

In those days, we were taught to lower your head and drill the top of your helmet into the running back's chest. Repeatedly running into things with the top of your head might cause some compression of the cervical vertebrae.

For many years, I was plagued with pain in my neck. I visited my general practitioner and a couple of orthopedic doctors. They took numerous X-rays and assured me that my neck vertebrae were compressed and that I clearly needed surgery to "fix" this problem. I said no. So, they offered me pain medication and muscle relaxers.

Years later, one of my friends suggested that I visit a chiropractor. I was leery about alternative medicine, but I felt I had nothing to lose. The chiropractor told me that I was indeed in bad shape, and I needed to see him three times per week for six months. Even then, he said that we might not be able to make significant improvement.

If you are unfamiliar with chiropractic adjustments, they work something like this. You lie on a table, and the chiropractor palpates your spine, looking for a vertebra that is out of alignment. (They are supposed to be aligned one above the other.) When the chiropractor finds a rebellious vertebra, he or she then asks you to relax. Then the chiropractor twists or pushes the vertebra back toward where it is supposed to be. (There is usually a crunching or popping noise when this happens.)

Your vertebrae function better when they are mobile. If one of them is out of alignment, then it is quite often because it is no longer able to move well. Therefore, the chiropractor is moving the vertebra for you.

On the downside, after six months of three-times-per-week adjustments, I had significantly less money. But on the upside, the painful neck episodes were down to twice a year instead of once per month. I was thankful that I had been introduced to the benefits of chiropractic adjustment, and I continued to see my chiropractor once every month or two for a few more years.

When I began practicing the self-directed, brain-based mobility training taught in the Z-Health R-Phase certification, things changed rather quickly. These drills include neck rotation, lateral flexion, glides, and the like. In other words, I began to consciously move the individual vertebrae of my neck on a regular basis. If we maintain the mobility of our cervical vertebrae, then they are unlikely to get "stuck" in a position that is out of alignment.

Here's how my paradigm changed. I thought I had a permanent neck injury. (The doctors and their X-rays confirmed this.) Chiropractic adjustments helped reduce the frequency of the painful episodes and that was wonderful. However, when I started moving each of the vertebrae in my neck, I improved the range of motion of my head and neck, and the painful episodes completely disappeared. I was able to cause positive adaptive changes in my neck structure. I shifted the responsibility for the care and maintenance of my neck from the medical system and my chiropractor to *myself*. If I move all the vertebrae in my neck, then my neck remains mobile and pain free. It is my job to do this.

I am constantly adapting to exactly what I am doing whether or not I want to. This is unavoidable. If I want to improve my mobility, then I must spend time practicing quality movements. And the unavoidable truth is that no one can do this for me.

Chapter 2: You Are Not a Collection of Body Parts

If it should happen that someone falls on your knee and damages its ligaments, then you would probably go to the emergency room, and a knee doctor (in other words, an orthopedic surgeon) would likely visit you there. And fortunately, in America, we have exceptional knee surgeons. One of them will do some work on your knee while you are asleep, and hopefully you will wake up and begin your journey toward a complete recovery with a fully functional knee. An even more dramatic version of this same story would have you visiting the doctor with a severely arthritic, bone-on-bone, painful, and nonfunctioning knee. The anesthesiologist would put you under, and the orthopedic surgeon would remove portions of your leg bones and give you shiny titanium and plastic replacements. You might awaken and be once again pain free. I feel very fortunate to have this level of medical care available to me here in America.

Unfortunately, knowing that these stories are commonplace leads us to believe that the knee is an independent body part that can be broken and repaired or removed, discarded, and replaced. This is somewhat true. However, the knee is not really a separate body part but is rather integral to the brain/body system. When you replace a knee, you change the way the system functions.

If your foot and ankle are not properly functioning, then this can cause a suboptimal performance pattern to exist at the knee. For example, take someone with flat feet or feet turned outward or someone who is bowlegged. These positions will not permit the knee to function as it was designed to function. Over time, you may develop a chronic pain experience that might show up as pain in the knee. Conversely, if the knee is not functioning properly or you have had your knee replaced, then your hip may suffer. Remember that there is usually acute pain associated with a traumatic injury as when someone falls on your knee. Chronic pain is different and can be the result of inefficient movement patterns that you have been carrying around with you for a long time. Acute pain and chronic pain are very different animals. We will look into pain more deeply in chapter 5.

The Body

We have a no return policy on our body, yet most people treat it quite badly. We can learn to perform amazing athletic feats with this body or to play beautiful melodies on a wide variety of musical instruments. Yet many people have not achieved even a portion of their athletic potential, or they are living a less than rewarding life and suffering with debilitating, chronic pain.

Imagine, if you will, that these people are drinking, smoking, eating fast food, and sitting around enjoying the comforts of their recliners and their wide-screen TVs. Day after day, their bodies are declining. When they one day wake up and discover they are overweight, have health issues, move very poorly, and have chronic pain, they are taken completely by surprise: "I didn't do anything. How did I get injured?" This is not an injury. This is a very important point to acknowledge as we undergo our paradigm shift. Chronic pain does not mean that you have an injury. The brain/body system is functioning poorly, and there is an associated pain experience because you are no longer athletic.

"But I have pain, so I must have an injury. I am confused because I don't remember injuring myself."

How did we end up with this way of looking at things? We became convinced during our childhood that the doctors and the medical system exist to help us both repair and take care of our bodies. This is similar to the way we view the car we drive. We drive it until it breaks and then we take it to the repair shop, and they fix it. A qualified mechanic must perform any maintenance done on this vehicle.

It is quite easy to see how this has happened. Whenever we became ill as children, our parents took us to the doctor. The doctor gave us a pile of unidentifiable magic pills, our symptoms improved, and eventually we were all well again. Why did we get sick in the first place? Of course, we didn't know. The doctors attributed it to microbes, bacteria, viruses, or other infinitesimally small things that we couldn't see. But it certainly wasn't our fault, and we became *convinced* that we would not have regained our health without the doctor's assistance.

The care, maintenance, and repair of our body really are not the doctor's jobs but rather *ours*. Many people in other cultures and other times have lived healthy, active, energetic lives and enjoyed a pain-free old age. Surely, some of these folk were lucky and were genetically blessed. However, physical activity was much more common in those eras and cultures without computers, video games, desk jobs, and cars. In addition, some people learned to listen to their bodies and therefore were more in tune with what was necessary to maintain their health. We had to listen to our bodies when we could not transfer the responsibility for their care to our doctor.

When I first began traveling to Russia, I was amazed to find what was in my friends' refrigerators: a huge variety of herbs and natural remedies. What was this all about? They could not count on the Russian medical system to "fix" them. They knew that they were responsible for their own health. So, they learned which herbs reduced blood pressure, which foods kept their digestive system regular, and which ointments to use for rashes and bites. They did not rush to the doctor at every drop of the hat.

One of the flaws in the way we Americans see things is that we often believe that it is the doctor's job to ensure that we are healthy and live a long, pain-free life. Another of the flaws in our paradigm is that our body is a separate entity and that we are free to abuse it. After all, there are many kinds of doctors and an increasingly amazing medical system that can and will fix whatever damage we do. There are many doctors who are quite eager to replace your body parts when they no longer function as they should. This further reinforces the concept that our body is separate from who we really are and that the doctors can repair it. We do have a wondrous medical system. Americans have access to the most advanced technology for replacing damaged parts. America is undoubtedly the very best place on earth to be if you have a traumatic injury. The emergency teams can save your life, and the surgeons can put you back together. I want to be clear that I am not talking badly about the medical system or the doctors. But as doctors have become better and better at solving our health problems, we have become more and more insistent that our health is *their* responsibility.

> *Healthy people move well. Your movement quality is a skill. Primary responsibility for this skill lies with you.*

The last five years of my father's life were very unpleasant. His quality of life was poor. In his early years, he had been one of the strongest men I have ever seen. He was active and enjoyed life. When this was taken away, he was quite naturally depressed. In the end, he was miserable, but the medical system kept putting him back together so that he could suffer for another week, month, or year. Our medical system is absolutely the very best at preventing or delaying death. In fact, as the American population ages, this is really the primary function of our medical system — to help prevent or delay the inevitability of death. This is different than having good health and an excellent quality of life. For my father, death was an escape from a life that had become torture.

My father's story is not a unique one. I know many people who are living with excruciating, chronic pain. Not all of them are old. And our medical system appears to be ill-equipped to deal with this problem. Along with this reduced quality of life often comes hopelessness and despair. Increasingly larger doses of pain medications will not solve this problem.

We are going to die. This sad fact is one we don't want to face. Part of this is cultural and comes from our concept of living happily ever after. In some other cultures, they accept the inevitability of death and conduct their lives accordingly, enjoying and savoring each moment of their time here. Americans generally don't believe (or at least they hope) this time will ever come. And it is apparently the doctor's job to postpone this inevitability for as long as possible.

The real question should be: "How do we want to live?" We can be mobile, energetic, vibrant, intelligent, and athletic at any age. The first step to achieving this is to stop breaking ourselves and hoping the doctors can fix us. We must take responsibility for the body we have been given. We must take positive steps to make ourselves better. This is the *science of hope*. Your body is miraculously adaptive. You can make it stronger, more flexible, and more athletic if that is something you desire; you make a plan to achieve it, and you begin working on that plan. Just like you learned to read, write, and talk, you can learn to move better. And as you learn to move better, your body will begin to change. As you begin to change your body and become more athletic, you will develop a more positive view of yourself and your world.

The Mind

Just like we often view the body as someone else's responsibility, a separate thing that we can break and fix and break and fix at will, the responsibility for our minds has been handed over to others. When we were children, we were shipped off to school. There, the teachers (who no doubt had our best interests at heart) stuffed our heads with the important things that would help us make it through life. We were taught math, science, language, geography, and history. The teachers told us to sit still, be quiet, and pay attention. Physical activity, if there was any, was relegated to physical education classes or recess breaks. It seems that children move less and less each year during the school day.

We seem to be trying to separate movement from the development of the mind. Movement actually helps strengthen the neural pathways of the brain and enhances the higher order thought processes. Here is a recommendation: if you want people to pay attention, then give them frequent breaks and have them move around. This is especially important with children, where the attention span is naturally quite short. (Actually, we adults are not really much better at paying attention for long periods of time.)

Once again, I am not talking badly about our educational system. America produces exceptional mathematicians, physicists, geologists, engineers, musicians, doctors, astronauts, and more. It is commendable that we pass on this knowledge to schoolchildren and young adults. And as we amass more and more technical knowledge, we are forced to pack more and more information into their heads. Adults and children are better equipped than ever to handle the challenges of our high-tech world.

But our minds are not separate from our bodies. Schoolteachers are not responsible for all the mental skills we have. Math, history, and science are important, and their study improves our reasoning abilities. But these subjects will not help us fall down gracefully, climb a tree, or avoid an oncoming bicycle. The development of quality movement skills is essential to our physical well-being, but it is also important for the creation of neural pathways inside the brain. These neural connections, created by our movements, improve our cognitive abilities. Hopefully, the use of our brain does not stop upon graduation. Therefore, as adults, we should look for new mental challenges, and we should continue to try to improve our movement skills. We should assume some responsibility for the care, maintenance, and development of what goes on inside our heads.

It seems that there is an increasing, national problem with attention deficit disorder or some variant of this diagnosis. This problem can be created or exacerbated by lack of exercise and poor movement skills. The incidence of attention deficit disorder is rivaled only by the prevalence of depression in our society. For both of these inconveniences, we once again rely on the medical community and the pharmaceutical companies. The reason we have attention deficit disorder and depression is because our society has a deficiency of Ritalin and Prozac. Certainly, we could not change what is going on inside our heads without these drugs. Or could we?

We all have voices inside our heads. When we are "in the present" and practice quality movement skills with focus, we can quiet these voices. Therefore, movement practice can be a form of meditation. This is a significant part of martial arts and yoga practice. They are designed to help us become calmer and more centered and to reduce our stress. They also help reduce the inner dialogue. Physical play and sports activities provide similar benefits. While we are fully engaged in our play, we are having fun, and our mental self-talk quiets down a bit. Remember to find time in your life for some play. Your quality of life will be much higher.

The brain has lots of jobs. Much of the stuff we are taught in school helps us with the skill of memory and helps us develop problem-solving abilities. But the brain is responsible for a lot more than just finding the correct answers for tests. The brain controls the movement of virtually all the muscles in the body. But it must have a good feedback mechanism if this control is to work properly. This means to move our arm well, we must know how far, how fast, and with how much force we are moving it. This is called *proprioceptive feedback,* and it comes from the processing of sensory inputs from our limbs. Quality movement practice reinforces the neural pathways of these proprioceptive feedback loops. This is another case of the use-it-or-lose-it rule. We will come back to this concept again and again. If you want to develop or maintain quality movement skills, then you must ask your body to perform quality movement skills. If you do not do this, then you will lose these skills and develop poor movement patterns filled with compensations and inefficiencies.

In addition to schoolwork, muscular contractions, and feedback from your proprioceptive sensory system, your brain must handle two other significant sensory input systems: the vestibular system (or inner ear) and the vision system. It is the high-quality integration of the proprioceptive, vestibular, and visual systems that combine to give us balance. For an excellent, in-depth look at how these systems work together, check out Scott McCredie's book, *Balance: In Search of the Lost Sense.*[6]

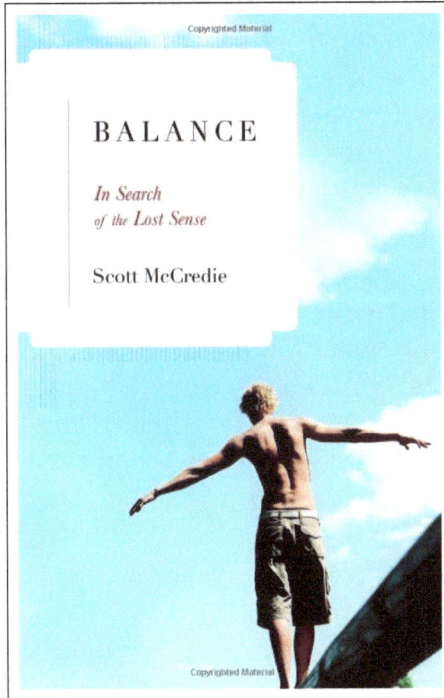

The vestibular system, our inner ear, is responsible for providing the brain with information about where is up and where we are going. Even with your eyes closed, you will know which way is up. When the car begins to move, you are aware that you are accelerating and that you are going somewhere. When you were a child, you loved to stimulate your vestibular system. This is why you wanted to spend time on a swing or turn around in circles until you fell down. This is an essential part of our childhood development. This developmental phase should not be skipped.

---

[6] Scott McCredie, *Balance: In Search of the Lost Sense* (New York: Little, Brown, 2007).

What happens when you become an adult in twenty-first-century America? You never turn around in circles again. You never swing on a swing. You never roll down a grass-covered hill. You stop playing, having fun, and stimulating your vestibular system. As a result, you may find that you don't move well anymore. For many people, simply turning around to see what is behind them causes an uncomfortable sensation of dizziness. They risk losing their balance and falling down.

We need the ability to turn around so that we can avoid danger. It is just one of the requirements for quality athletic movement skills. Without accurate processing of the signals from your inner ear, and without knowing where up is and where you are going, it simply may no longer be safe for you to move. Regularly challenging our vestibular system is the best way to maintain its function or to regain it.

The third and most powerful of the sensory input systems is the visual system. Isn't it amazing that we can take in so much information through our eyes? The images from both of our eyes are compared within the brain and used to construct a real-time, three-dimensional representation of the world around us. And our brain is doing this all the time we are awake! How much computer processing would it take to do that?

This system allows us to focus directly on objects and to know what is around us through our peripheral vision field. It lets us perceive movement and judge how far away an object is or how fast it is approaching us. But, hypothetically speaking, suppose we spent all day, every day staring at a computer screen or texting on our iPhone. We would probably become really good at texting, using a mouse, and reading the fine print under the icons on our monitor. But what would happen to our athletic vision skills? Would we be able to track a rapidly moving object with our eyes or change focal length? No. We would begin to lose these abilities.

There are six extraocular muscles surrounding each eye that control its movement up and down and left and right. There are other muscles that change the focus of the eyes from near to far. These muscles, like all muscles, require regular use in order to keep them functioning properly. Texting on your smartphone simply will not improve your vision or maintain the ability to rapidly track objects in space. And if your vision is compromised, then it will interfere with quality movement skills.

> *Vision is the highest priority sensory input system. Therefore, we must regularly challenge our vision skills.*

On a regular basis, we must maintain and challenge all our sensory input systems: our proprioception, vestibular, and visual systems. This is how we will keep the brain sharp and functioning at its peak. Practicing quality movement skills is the key to this maintenance.

The System

The brain and the body are supposed to work together as a team. The ancient Hindu and Chinese philosophies say that there should be a balance between the mind and the body. Do you agree? Just like we can have muscle imbalances, the brain/body system can also be out of balance.

At one point in my life, I was starting a new business. I worked at a desk doing intense mental work for more than eighty hours per week. You could say that I was motivated, driven, determined, and very dedicated. Unfortunately, after several months of this effort, I found that I was unable to go to sleep at night. Fortunately, I didn't run to the doctor for sleeping pills. Instead, I listened to the brain/body system. Mine was completely out of whack. At night, my brain was tired, but my body wasn't. I was getting little or no physical exercise. No wonder I couldn't sleep. And since I didn't sleep well, I couldn't think well during the day. So, I drank more coffee and worked more hours. This was a vicious circle. Finally, I began to exercise more regularly again. Once I resumed my exercise program, I felt better, slept better, and was more productive at work. Physical activity was an essential (and missing) part for my continued health and well-being.

There are a couple of important lessons in this story. First, if we listen to the brain/body system, then we can very often learn what we need to do to improve how we perform and how we feel. Second, notice that the responsibility for this change was mine — not the doctor's and not the medical system's.

All movement is a joint effort of the brain and body. The brain creates an image or prediction of what the movement will be; signals are sent to the various muscles throughout the body; sensory input from the proprioceptive, vestibular, and visual systems are processed and evaluated throughout the duration of the movement; and then the actual performance is compared with the desired, visualized movement. From this, we learn how our bodies move, how to better sequence our movements, and what it feels like when we perform certain movements. This allows the brain to construct better, clearer three-dimensional movies of our movement repertoire. This also helps the brain plot out and create new movement patterns or sequences that we might not have done before.

If we are not challenging our brain/body system with complex and quality physical movements, then we are not using a large and important portion of our brain, and we are not stimulating the wide variety of sensory input systems associated with those movements. As a result, our ability to move will decline. The brain, the peripheral nervous system, and the muscles and fascia of the body require frequent use. All these systems will degrade over time if they are not used.

Takeaway

We are responsible for improving our minds and bodies. The schools and the medical system are wonderful, but they are not in charge of all maintenance and repair of this system. This is good news. We are not solely dependent on them for our future well-being, and we are far from helpless. If your mental skills or your movement abilities aren't what you want them to be, then you can change them. We are amazingly adaptable and can evolve to be better through our own efforts.

If we learn to listen to our brain and body, then they will provide us with information about what they want. This knowledge will allow us to get a little bit better every day. More is not always necessarily better. Working out really hard can be good for you, or it can break you. We are looking for just the right dosage that will make us better.

The brain and the body work together as one highly integrated and interdependent system. As a result, a change in one part of the system does have an effect on other, seemingly unrelated parts of the system. This is where the Z-Health brain-centric training paradigm might begin to seem strange. You might have a pain in your right ankle. Performing vision drills or focused wrist mobility exercises might cause your pain to disappear. Is this a trick? No, it is not. Everything is connected together and integrated by the central nervous system.

> *Since the brain and body form one integrated system, anything can cause anything.*

Paradigm Shift

If you have been involved at any time with organized sports, then your coach has probably pushed you on occasion. We cannot get stronger unless we exert intense effort at least some of the time. We cannot improve our endurance if all we do is talk about it. Therefore, early on, I learned that working out harder would make you better. Guaranteed. Or so I thought.

As a Tae Kwon Do instructor, I routinely pushed the class hard. More kicks would make them better at kicking. More stretching would make them more flexible.

When I started The Kettlebell Club, I brought with me the same mentality. The students would get stronger if they lifted heavier weights, and their endurance would increase if we did more kettlebell swings. And I pushed myself right along with the students.

What I observed over the first five years was that clients would get stronger and then most of them would develop injuries or pain. I was constantly watching their form and ensuring that they weren't at risk of injury. But they still ended up in pain. This made me very unhappy. My job was to help my clients move better, be stronger, be healthier, and have a better life. My job was not to cause them injury or pain.

Here's the paradigm shift that I made. Working out hard can make you better, or it can break you. It all depends on the individual and his or her current movement skills and fitness level. Exercise is like a drug. Too little will not help, and too much can kill you. We need to find the correct amount to cause a positive outcome. The precise amount is specific to the individual. What is good for me may be too much for you and vice versa.

Complex movement skills involve the use of the entire brain/body system. If we push too hard on the system, then the brain can give us fatigue, poor movement skills, or pain. Our complex movement patterns will tend to break down when too much load is applied. Structural damage can occur at the weakest point in the movement's kinetic chain. We are an integrated system of bones, muscles, tendons, and a complex nervous system that controls it all.

When we swing a kettlebell or lift other weights, we are applying a load to a movement skill. If the movement quality is not excellent, then we will further ingrain the poor movement skills and any compensations in those movement patterns. If we apply enough load or enough repetitions to an inefficient movement pattern, then we are likely to break.

Now I know that working out hard might make you better. Maybe. Or it might break you. Working out harder might mean that we need to spend more time working on our movement quality so that we can safely apply additional load.

Chapter 3: The Brain Is in Charge

The most important organ in your body is the brain. It controls nearly everything that goes on inside us humans. Of course, the brain allows us to think and to carry on an unending internal dialogue with ourselves. But this is not the primary function of our central nervous system.

The brain is constantly processing the information from our skin, muscles, joints, eyes, and balance systems. It is difficult to imagine the volume and variety of information being processed. Simultaneously, the brain is controlling functions such as posture, muscular contractions, body temperature, blood pressure, heart rate, digestion, and much more. The brain is in charge of this system and is constantly accepting input, evaluating it, and processing it, and then creating outputs such as desires, feelings, and movements.

According to John Medina in his book *Brain Rules*:

> The brain appears to be designed to (1) solve problems (2) related to surviving (3) in an unstable outdoor environment, and (4) to do so in nearly constant motion.[7]

I like this description. He mentions problem solving, survival, adaptability, and movement. Each of these is an important function of the brain. We will look further at the reasons we have a brain in this chapter.

The Purpose of the Brain
In many ways, the function of our brains is similar to that of animal brains—maintaining bodily functions, seeking to reproduce, and finding sustenance. Brains are used to process sensory inputs, to help us to escape danger, and to

---

[7] John Medina, *Brain Rules: 12 Principles for Surviving and Thriving at Work, Home, and School* (Seattle: Pear Press, 2014), 4.

continue our existence and the existence of our species. Human brains also include a larger cerebral cortex than animals and that gives us the ability to think, to be creative, and to be self-aware. The evolutionary process has encased this amazing brain in a container of bone to protect it from injury. It is not only important but also essential. We are looking for insight into how we can improve ourselves. So, we must ask the question, "What is the purpose of the brain?" The brain serves three primary functions: prediction, movement, and survival.

Prediction

One of the reasons we have brains is so we can predict the future. Imagine that you asked to borrow someone's car, and your friend tosses you the car keys. You respond by predicting the future while the keys are in flight.

In the world of physics, there are complex equations to describe the motion of the keys as they float through the air. The keys have a mass, there is wind resistance, and the effect of gravity is pulling the keys back down to planet earth. All these factors can be input into some mathematical formula and the trajectory of the keys computed. Fortunately, we don't need to do this. We see the keys flying through the air, and we are able to instantaneously predict where the keys will be when they reach our hands. We are really good at this difficult bit of computation, and we can predict the future position of external bodies in motion.

But look at what we did with our hand as the keys were flying toward us. We quickly began moving to put our hand in the place where the keys would be. To do this, we had to predict the amount of complex muscular contractions required to bend our elbow to the correct angle, take a slight step to the right, and rotate our wrist so that our palm was facing upward. Amazingly, we did this without any conscious thought.

Movement, in fact, is really about prediction. Most of the time, we do not move with any conscious thought. You will find that conscious thought usually interferes with quality athletic movement and causes our movements to be more tense, slower, and much less fluid. In this example, we predicted that we would move in a way that would allow us to catch the keys. We don't know how we moved to do this. We don't remember whether we were inhaling or exhaling. We didn't plan to turn our head slightly and track the keys with our eyes. Everything that occurred in our movement sequence happened automatically in response to our prediction of the future event that we "had already moved" in a certain way.

The way we perceive the world around us is also based on prediction. According to Jeff Hawkins, author of *On Intelligence*:

> *Our brains use stored memories to constantly make predictions about everything we see, feel, and hear...The vast majority of predictions occur outside of awareness...Prediction is so pervasive that what we "perceive" – that is, how the world appears to us – does not come solely from our senses. What we perceive is a combination of what we sense and of our brain's memory-derived predictions.*[8]

---

[8] Jeff Hawkins, *On Intelligence*, With Sandra Blakeslee (New York: Henry Holt, 2004), 86–7.

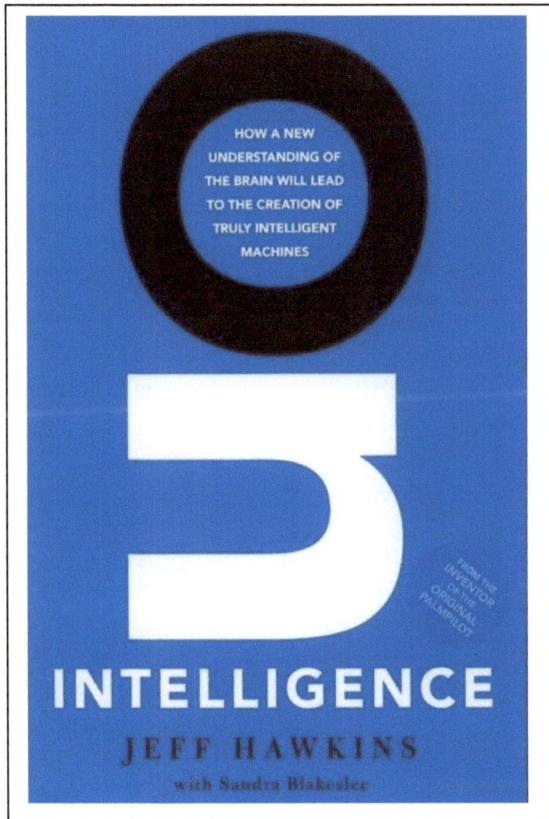

HOW A NEW
UNDERSTANDING OF
THE BRAIN WILL LEAD
TO THE CREATION OF
TRULY INTELLIGENT
MACHINES

ON
INTELLIGENCE

JEFF HAWKINS

with Sandra Blakeslee

FROM THE INVENTOR OF THE ORIGINAL PALMPILOT

What he is saying is that we don't see with only our eyes. We predict what we should see and use our vision to improve on or alter our prediction. This is one of the reasons why "eyewitness accounts" at crime scenes are so unreliable — we don't rely only on what information reached our eyes to determine what we think we saw.

Let's look at another example. Imagine you are returning home after a day at work. When you unlock your front door and enter your home, your eyes receive input about everything in the room. Most of this information is compared with the predicted or expected state of affairs, and if it meets your expectations, then it is ignored. The visual information we constantly receive would be overwhelming if we were forced to think about or consciously process all of it. Therefore, the brain compares ongoing visual information with stored memories and, based on predictions, only sends exception data (or things that are unexpected) to our consciousness for processing. In this example, we enter our home and notice there is a set of car keys lying on the table. This is unusual. What is that? Answer: car keys. Whose keys are these? Answer: the keys I loaned to Cousin Fred. Where is the car? I didn't see it in the driveway. And so on. Notice that we did not "see" all the other things in the room that were exactly as they were supposed to be.

> *One of the primary functions of the brain is prediction.*

Movement

Another function of the brain is the support of movement. Animals have brains and are mobile, while plants have no brains and are not free to roam around. It seems that wherever we find a brain, we find it exists in a biological construct that moves. The argument can be made, therefore, that the primary function of the brain is to support movement.

In his excellent TED Talk, "The Real Reason for Brains," Dr. Daniel Wolpert argues this very fact.[9] He uses the sea squirt as an example. The sea squirt is a marine invertebrate that begins its life as a tadpole-like creature. It swims around for one or two days and then affixes itself to a rock. Once it has found its new home on the rock, it undergoes a metamorphosis that includes, among other things, the digestion of its own brain. Since it no longer has

---

[9] "The Real Reason for Brains," Daniel Wolpert, TED Talk, Filmed July 2011, http://www.ted.com/talks/daniel_wolpert_the_real_reason_for_brains.

any need to move around, it doesn't need a brain. It has no need to provide food and energy for such a high-maintenance organ. Now, the sea squirt hangs out on the rock in a blissful, brain-free state and waits for food to pass by. (I know quite a few people who aspire to this state.)

We have brains that plan our movements, and we use our output nerves to cause our muscles to contract. In addition, we have other nerves that provide feedback about the location of our body parts and other information regarding the external world. Our brains process signals from our input nerves, or afferent nerves, and then other signals are transmitted on our output nerves, or efferent nerves. As we learned to move better and to develop dexterity and more complicated movement skills, our brains continued to evolve, and we were able to plan our movement strategies better. We required larger brains in order to develop these more challenging movement patterns and to better predict the incredible variety of patterns in our ever-changing world. In this way of looking at the purpose of the brain, we first learned to move, we developed larger and more complex brains, and then as a result, we morphed into sentient, planning, emotional, and introspective creatures.

> *The only reason we have a brain may be to support movement.*

Survival

Certainly at the top of the list of the many functions or purposes of the brain is survival. Humans, like all other creatures, have an instinct for survival. We will do nearly anything to ensure our own survival, the survival of our children, and the continuation of our species. This is one of the highest priorities of our brain. If you are stranded outside during a blizzard, then you will begin to get very cold. Sensing this drop in body temperature, the brain will do everything it can to protect your organs and ensure your survival, even at the expense of letting your hands and feet freeze.

The human brain is also a self-centered and greedy organ. It wants you to survive, but the brain itself comes first. That is not a bad thing. It really is a rather important organ.

> *Although the brain represents only 2% of the body weight, it receives 15% of the cardiac output and consumes 20% of the total body oxygen.*[10]

The brain also voraciously uses about 20 percent of the calories we consume.[11] The brain wants blood, energy, and oxygen for itself.

Since the brain is concerned with your survival and its own continued existence, it encourages you to do things like eat more because it can't be sure when you will find food again. This is not particularly helpful if you are on a diet and trying to lose weight by restricting your caloric intake. Similarly, your brain tells you that you should not exercise because this burns calories you might need when running away from predators. According to the brain, you should probably spend more time lounging around in the shade of a big tree and snacking on delicious food.

Eating food and getting enough rest are both important to the brain, but there are other things the brain desires, since it is concerned with our survival. For example, we need to be able to find food and to avoid danger. We might need a good memory and the ability to reason in order to find our

---

[10] Vasha Jain, Michael C. Langham, and Felix W. Wehrli, "MRI Estimation of Global Brain Oxygen Consumption Rate," *Journal of Cerebral Blood Flow and Metabolism* 30, no. 9 (2010): 1598–607.
[11] Covián F. Grande, "Energy Metabolism of the Brain in Children," *Anales Espanoles de Pediatria* 12, no. 3 (1979): 235–44.

next meal. We probably need clear vision, good hearing, quick reflexes, and functional movement skills in order to avoid animal attacks, falling rocks, or angry neighbors. These things might cause us bodily harm and threaten our survival. In other words, your body and its exceptional athletic abilities are very important to the brain. In order for you to survive in this harsh and cruel world, you must be strong, quick, and agile, and you must be able to think well. Your brain will become unhappy if any of these abilities begin to decline. The brain will be less able to ensure your survival, and it will try to communicate its unhappiness to you through some nonverbal message.

The purpose or function of the brain may be a prediction of how an object falls or knowing how the world around us is expected to appear. Or it may be to support our complex movement skills and the development of new ones. But absolutely, 100 percent for sure, the first priority of our brain is to ensure our survival. These are all the same things, and I will refer to them interchangeably. Our predictive abilities and the acquisition of new and amazing movement skills are both elements contained within the brain's primary purpose of survival. We must be able to predict how the path to our garden will look so that we will notice the snake lying in wait for us. We must be able to move well, stop quickly, make an evaluation, and create a new travel plan. Predicting, planning, reacting, and moving are all ways our brain helps to ensure our survival.

Our brains will go to great lengths to ensure our survival. And if we do things to help the brain achieve its goal, then it will reward us in many ways, such as with clearer thinking, better memory, improved balance, more energy, greater strength, and increased endurance.

> *The primary function of the brain is to*
> *ensure our survival.*

Brain Maps

As long ago as the 1930s, scientists had discovered that physical representations of our bodies exist inside our brains. There are maps for our hands, our lips, our feet, and all other parts of our bodies. In a surgical procedure pioneered by Dr. Wilder Penfield, electrodes were used to stimulate various areas of the brain in patients who were awake during their brain surgery procedures. This was made possible by the fact that the brain itself has no pain receptors. As various places were stimulated, patients were asked if they felt anything. Patients would indicate that they felt a tingling in their left ring finger or their nose. After nearly two decades and more than five hundred patients, Penfield published his findings in 1950 in a book called *The Cerebral Cortex of Man*.[12]

What this book revealed is that a corresponding physical map in the brain represents each body part. Furthermore, the size of each of these maps is related to the quality and quantity of the sensory input from that area. As an example, the hands and the lips are very sensitive and are able to quickly differentiate small objects. These highly innervated body parts have comparatively large maps in the brain.[13]

> *Each of your body parts is represented*
> *by a physical brain map.*

---

[12] Wilder Penfield and Theodore Rasmussen, *The Cerebral Cortex of Man* (New York: Macmillan, 1950).
[13] Sandra Blakeslee and Matthew Blakeslee, *The Body Has a Mind of Its Own: How Body Maps in Your Brain Help You Do (Almost) Everything Better* (New York: Random House, 2007), 15–20.

If you are interested in reading more about brain maps, I suggest Sandra Blakeslee and Matthew Blakeslee's book, *The Body Has a Mind of Its Own*.[14]

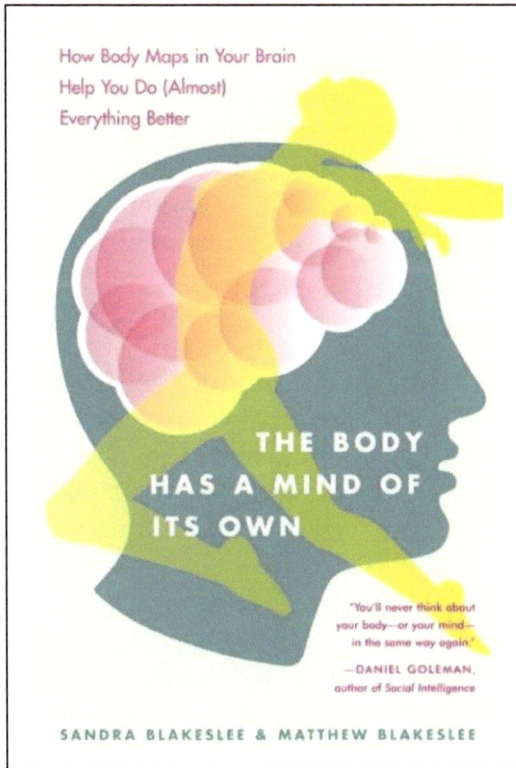

Michael Merzenich built on Penfield's work and discovered that not only did the brain hold physical representations of our body but also that these brain maps were constantly changing.[15] If you stop using a body part, then the associated brain map will become fuzzy and unclear and begin to shrink in size. By contrast, if you were to take up violin or piano and practice diligently,

---

[14] Ibid.

[15] Norman Doidge, *The Brain That Changes Itself: Stories of Personal Triumph from the Frontiers of Brain Science* (New York: Penguin Books, 2007), 45–65.

then the maps of your fingers will become more clearly defined and increase in size.

For many years, scientists were certain that the brain developed through adolescence and into early adulthood and then its structure became fixed. There was a part of the brain that felt the left hand and a part of the brain that controlled the movement of the left hand. If these parts of the brain were injured, then you would simply no longer have movement or sensation in your left hand. It was believed that the damage was permanent, and there was no hope for recovery.

We now know that this is untrue.

Edward Taub was able to demonstrate that many stroke victims are able to regain the use of their afflicted limbs and reacquire normal or near-normal movement. How is this possible? What Taub learned was that when a portion of the brain was damaged by a stroke, the associated map can be damaged. This can cause a loss of the ability to move or feel a body part such as an arm and a hand. But the brain has the ability to rewire itself and to use other, nondamaged areas of the brain to create and hold a new map. Stroke victims are not destined to live out their lives hopelessly facing the inability to function.

This work of learning to use the afflicted body part, and it is work, is quite difficult. It is similar to learning to use your body the first time when you were a child. Perhaps it is even more difficult because the brain is much more malleable in our youth. But it can be done. If the patient is dedicated and works hard enough, then the brain will construct a new map, and the patient can relearn lost movement skills.[16]

---

[16] Doidge, *The Brain That Changes Itself*, 137–57.

You are not stuck with remaining exactly as you are. You can become much more if that is your desire. The brain is plastic or changeable. One of the terms for the brain's ability to restructure itself is *neuroplasticity*. This has dramatic implications for each of us. We can learn new physical skills and acquire new memories throughout our lives. With each passing day, we can become better by challenging our brain. Similarly, a failure to provide adequate stimulus to the brain will cause its function to steadily decline.

> *Your brain maps are constantly changing as a result of your movements and experiences.*

Norman Doidge has written an enlightening and very readable book on the subject of neuroplasticity, *The Brain That Changes Itself.*[17] It is inspirational to hear how people have recovered from what was once thought to be hopeless brain injuries.

---

[17] Ibid.

"The power of positive thinking finally gains scientific credibility. Mind-bending, miracle-making, reality-busting stuff...Straddles the gap between science and self-help."–The New York Times

THE
BR IN
THAT CHANGES
ITSELF

Stories of Personal Triumph From
the Frontiers of Brain Science

NORMAN DOIDGE, M.D.

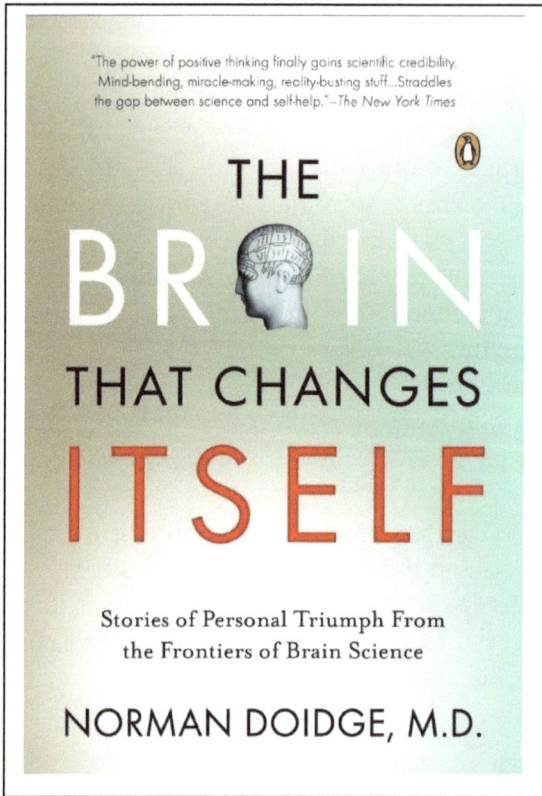

So, we have maps in our brains. And a loss of sensory input quality will cause a reduction in map quality or map clarity. What can we do with this information? We can apply this to the most important function of the brain in order to ensure our survival. If our brain maps are fuzzy or unclear, then the brain knows less about the outside world. This threatens our ability to survive. In addition, our movement quality is dependent on sensory input so that we know how to move well and so that we can more clearly predict the outcome of our movements. Cloudy or unclear sensory-movement maps cause our brain stress because this threatens our survival. Threats make the brain unhappy. When the brain is happy, it will reward us with increased strength, better balance, and improved athleticism. When the brain is unhappy, it will try to communicate that to us too. To do this, the brain may limit our range of motion, make us seem uncoordinated, decrease our reaction time, make us tired, or cause us to experience pain.

Could the chronic pain in your shoulder be the result of a cloudy, unclear sensory map? Yes, it could. Could you make the brain happy by clarifying your sensory-movement maps, and could that reduce your pain? Yes, it is possible.

> *Cloudy or unclear brain maps are a threat to the brain/body system.*

Skill Development

We can increase the clarity of our brain maps through focused quality movements. This activity will cause the brain to undergo physiological changes, increasing the number and quality of neural connections. Similarly, we can positively affect the brain's function through the creation of new memories and the development of new skills. Storing memories and acquiring new talents require focused work and utilize a lot of energy and are therefore challenging activities. However, it is very much worth the effort. Continuing to challenge our brains to learn new things encourages their proper function and helps to keep us young. We are not designed to stop learning when we leave school as young adults. Rather, we must continue to use our brains and to push them to acquire new skills throughout our lives. We must use it or lose it. And in case you hadn't noticed, the brain hates boredom. This is why television, books, and social media are so successful. These activities keep us from being bored. Unfortunately, our movement skills are not challenged when someone or something else does the entertaining for us. And many areas of the brain remain unchallenged while we are watching our favorite beer commercials.

As stated earlier, the brain is an organ that is hungry for fuel or energy and oxygen. But the brain also wants new experiences and stimulation. It wants you to play and to learn new skills. Play always involves exposure to novel things; otherwise, it ceases to be fun. Tic-tac-toe is fun at first but eventually becomes boring, since you know the outcome. Continue to find fun, fresh, and challenging activities to stimulate the brain. This will make the brain happy, and it will reward you.

> ### The brain craves novelty and challenge.

Unfortunately, most of what we do each day is done on autopilot. Sometimes, you will get into the car, start it, and begin driving without noticing that you have done all these things. "Where am I going? Oh yeah. Now I remember." (Okay, perhaps that is just *my* experience.) But this sort of autonomous behavior is a good thing. If we had to consciously think about *everything*, then we would be overwhelmed. Could we notice every aspect of the world around us? Certainly not! Are we able to pay attention to every feeling and sensation coming into our body through our hands, feet, and other body parts? Could we consciously control the activities of each and every muscle in our bodies as we opened the car door and sat down? No way.

But learning new skills requires us to do some version of this. We must focus on at least a portion of the task in a conscious manner. We must pay attention to the details in the beginning of our efforts to improve any talent. Then, as we get better and better at a particular skill, we can refine it. This will be made possible, since we won't need to consciously pay attention to the whole skill. Some of it will become automatic or habit. Then we can consciously focus on a new part of the skill.

Let's look at this process of new skill acquisition. According to the 1967 Fitts and Posner model of motor skill development, there are three distinct stages: cognitive, associative, and autonomous.[18]

During the *cognitive* stage, we must think about the skill we are trying to perform. As a result, the type of errors made are rather large, and usually the energy expenditure for our effort is excessive. We are rank amateurs during this stage, and we are learning what it is that we are trying to learn. As a result, although we are not very good at the skill, we can make progress very quickly. This is an exciting phase of the development. It is usually important to have qualified coaching during this period. We will remain in this stage for one thousand or more repetitions.

In the next stage of our skill development, the *associative* stage, we are doing a little better. The types of errors we are making are smaller. We don't need to think about every activity in detail. Our efficiency has improved. We are now able to identify many of our own mistakes. We have a very good idea about what we are trying to do, and we are learning to do it. Unfortunately, our progress slows down significantly. Portions of the activity are becoming repeatable. We will remain in this stage of development until we have completed between ten thousand and one hundred thousand repetitions.

The last stage of development is the *autonomous* stage. Now we perform the skill largely on autopilot. We are efficient, and the skill may appear effortless, using little or no unnecessary energy. Now we have much less requirement for cognitive input in order to perform the

---

[18] Paul Morris Fitts and Michael I. Posner, *Human Performance* (Belmont, CA: Brooks/Cole, 1967).

skill. As a result, we can focus on mental skills such as motivation and strategy. It can require more than one hundred thousand repetitions to reach this level of mastery.

> *Skill acquisition occurs in three stages: cognitive, associative, and autonomous.*

A few things are important about this skill acquisition process.

1. We must start all skill development in the cognitive stage where we actively think about and focus on what we are trying to do. Whether we are working on a new skill or trying to "rehabilitate" an existing skill, we must use focused, deliberate, and conscious practice in the beginning of the process.

2. We can develop a wide variety of new skills if we are willing to go through this difficult and lengthy process. Long-lasting skills cannot be acquired without diligent, repetitive, and focused practice. And no one can do this for us.

3. In the autonomous stage, we are performing skills essentially without conscious thought. If there are inefficient or compensatory actions in our autonomous skill, then we may not even know they exist, since these skills are most often performed outside our awareness. We must critically review our performance, and look for any areas that require correction.

Deliberate Practice

In the groundbreaking 1993 article, "The Role of Deliberate Practice in the Acquisition of Expert Performance," Dr. Anders Ericsson and his colleagues shared the results of their research into how we develop new talents.[19] After looking at many disciplines ranging from violin playing to playing chess to writing books, Ericsson et al. observed that two things are required to obtain an expert-level talent: regular deliberate practice and time. Specifically, they observed that two hours or more of daily, focused practiced over the course of ten years will most likely lead to the mastery of a talent. Ericsson and his colleagues correlated the ten years of focused study with the ten-thousand-hour rule. This rule states that it takes ten thousand hours of deep, deliberate practice to achieve mastery. Those who love what they do are more likely to practice alone and are willing to focus intently on this activity. Therefore, they are more likely to improve. This is not much of a surprise. What is surprising is the requirement of ten years or ten thousand hours to achieve this level. This is a lot of time and dedication.

Recall our discussion of myelin in chapter 1. This is the fatty, white, insulation-like material that is deposited on the outside of our neural circuitry when we regularly use it. This material improves the quality and speed of the electrical transmissions through our nervous system. This process of laying down myelin on our nerves takes time — lots of time. Putting down significant quantities of myelin can take thousands of repetitions, intense focus, and years of dedication. And as we get better, we can do new things, and we can get better at those things. Then we can learn new skills. An amateur cannot even practice movements that an accomplished person can do with ease. Few people can do what masters can do because they simply do not have the neurological wiring to do it. Our more advanced skills are built on our more elementary skills. And these

---

[19] K. Anders Ericsson, Ralf Th. Krampe, and Clemens Tesch-Romer, "The Role of Deliberate Practice in the Acquisition of Expert Performance," *Psychological Review* 100, no. 3 (1993): 363–406.

basic skills must be fast, accurate, and autonomous. This means that we must master the basics through relentless practice because it is on these skills that we develop the more advanced ones.

Whether it is the ability to play a piano or excel at chess, or physical skills such as throwing a football or pole vaulting, talent is not something that is exclusively a genetic gift. We are not born with exceptional talent. Experts in all fields must apply themselves diligently by spending thousands of hours practicing. We may be born with certain abilities, traits, or aptitudes that allow us the opportunity to excel at certain things. For example, a tall, lean, and extremely flexible young lady has some of the elements required to pursue a career in ballet. However, being tall, lean, and flexible does not mean you will be an exceptional ballet dancer. It does not mean you have balance, strength, and coordination. This occupation requires years of hard work, dedication, and practice.

We now know that everything is a skill, and we know how to obtain new skills. We must spend time in deep, deliberate practice, and we must persevere. Many years of practice will be required. But it would be much nicer if we could reduce the amount of time required to develop the new skills we desire. And we can do just that by ensuring we are practicing the right things at the right time and that we are fully engaged during our practice. These are the activities that will fire the right neural patterns, help us grow new dendrites on our nerve cells, and lay down myelin to improve our neural pathways.

> *Two keys to the development of skill mastery are regular, deep, deliberate practice and years of hard work.*

What is this *deliberate practice*? Here are some of the attributes of this special type of work toward the attainment of expert skills.

- It is designed specifically to improve performance.

- It can be repeated—a lot.

- Feedback on results is continuously available.

- It isn't much fun.

The reason for deep, deliberate practice is obvious—it works! However, in order to perform the work of regular, deep, deliberate practice, the athlete or artist must exhibit constant, relentless motivation or discipline. This motivation, like all skills, when practiced long enough, can become habit. The famous writer William Faulkner, author of *The Sound and the Fury* among others, was once asked if he wrote on a schedule or when he was inspired. He answered, "Of course, I only write when I am inspired. Fortunately, I am inspired at 9 o'clock each morning."

Neural Chunking

In chapter 1, I mentioned Daniel Coyle's book *The Talent Code*. In this book, Mr. Coyle says:

> *Skill consists of identifying important elements and grouping them into a meaningful framework. The name psychologists use for such organization is* chunking.[20]

This neural chunking is essential to skill mastery. This is what is clearly visible during the associative phase of our skill acquisition. As an example, let's look at how we develop the skill of reading. First, we learn to identify letters, numbers, punctuation, and other symbols. Then, we learn to identify words, and we associate meaning with those abstract representations. We practice over and over until the letters that form the word *cat* no longer mean c-a-t

---

[20] Coyle, *The Talent Code*, 77.

but rather correspond to an image of a furry domestic creature. This is chunking. Now, *cat* has a sound when it is pronounced and an underlying, associated meaning. When we see the word *cat*, we no longer need to read out the letters c-a-t. We have a neural chunk that represents this.

This neural chunking process morphs and improves so that it affects our ability to read phrases. The English language is especially full of phrases: "over the hill," "let the cat out of the bag," "in the blink of an eye," "throw caution to the wind," "run out of time," and the like. Once again, after we learn these phrases and their associated meanings, we establish a new neural chunk, and we no longer pay attention to the individual words in the expression. As we become more and more proficient at reading, we don't read letters or even all the words in each sentence. Take a look at this stream of characters:

Cn yu rd ths sntnc?

I bet it is not difficult for you. We use our chunks to infer meaning, and our predictive abilities allow us to anticipate the meaning of the sentence in advance.

All this is wonderful news! After we successfully acquire a new small skill, it is essentially downloaded into the preconscious area of our brain. We can access it, and we can use it, but we don't need to spend much energy or time "thinking" about it. We will be able to perform the skill faster. And it happens with less effort from the cerebral cortex (or our thinking brain). In fact, it happens so automatically that when we perform a complex movement, many pieces of the movement, these neural chunks, will take place completely outside our conscious thought process. An autonomous pattern is being created.

But what if the chunk contains some errors? How can we "fix" the chunk and improve our skill? The only way to fix neural chunks is to return to the beginning, to step one, consciously perform the skill, and create a new neural chunk, effectively overwriting the original chunk. This is difficult and tedious work. It may be more difficult than the creation of the original chunk. But there is no shortcut. In this way, we can refine our skills by breaking them down into their smallest components and looking for errors in the corresponding neural chunks. Then we can consciously and deliberately work to improve the quality of our movement by creating new and better chunks.

> *To fix errors in existing neural chunks, replace those chunks with new ones.*

Not all chunks are created equal. Some neural chunks are formed almost instantaneously, while others take much longer. Why does this happen? It would be good if we could find a secret formula that would allow us to create our desired neural chunks faster.

Imagine that you are a small child wandering around in the kitchen. Your mom is cooking dinner. You reach up to the stovetop because you are curious about what she is doing, and your hand touches the pot with the boiling soup above the open flame. Just as you do this, Mom sees you, panics, and shouts "No!" while grabbing for your little hand. You felt the heat from the fire, and you might have a slight burn from the pot, but in addition to this, there was a significant emotional context to the event. Mom was clearly upset, worried, and panicked, and you have never seen her move that fast.

How we feel greatly affects our ability to create new neural chunks. If you are not interested or you are not paying attention, then it will be difficult to cause the necessary adaptation in the nervous system. However, if you are excited, happy, curious, fascinated, or afraid, then new memories and chunks are formed more quickly and are more likely to be retained. These heightened emotional states are difficult to maintain; therefore, shorter and more frequent practice sessions are usually preferable to fewer and longer sessions.

As stated earlier, the brain detests boredom. Most highly skilled individuals truly love their practice and derive some joy from it. They may often see their sessions as fun. A love of practice combined with strict discipline is usually the only way to maintain the necessary focus required for deep, deliberate practice day after day and year after year.

> *Shorter and more frequent practice sessions will allow you to remain fresh and interested and create new neural chunks faster.*

Play

Just like people, animals have movement skills. Some of these abilities, as you likely know, are quite amazing. Have you ever seen a squirrel run along a power wire or jump from branch to branch and from tree to tree? How do they acquire these talents? Certainly, some of these skills are genetically inherited, but they also get lots of focused practice, since their survival depends on these skills. And fortunately for animals, they are not constantly distracted by abstract concepts, advertisements, forty-hour workweeks, and time-consuming obligations on social media. They are free to play, practice movement skills, eat, sleep, and repeat. It is not surprising that animals become quite proficient at their skills.

They begin developing their talents at a very young age. As soon as they are able to move about, they begin to play with their siblings. You have no doubt seen videos of baby lions or bear cubs fighting, nipping at one another, and wrestling in the grass. This is how they practice essential elements of their survival skills. Animals develop these abilities neither because they go to school nor because their parents make them do it. It is both interesting and fun. Because it is fun, the young animals are able to focus their attention for extended periods of time, an essential requirement for skill development.

Children and animals have something in common. They both love to play. Play is, by definition, fun. Play involves movement and creativity. It engages the body and mind. It is through play that we learn how to move, and we use this playtime to refine our skills. This is the original exercise — before we had to join a gym and to pay for the privilege of moving around. Play is nonthreatening, and we want this experience to go on and on. This is how children determine where their bodies are in three-dimensional space and how to improve their movement skills. They also learn what their limitations are in a relatively safe environment. What happened to fun and play? As we grew as children, we began to hear more and more statements like "Stop that! You are going to fall and hurt yourself." Of course, falling is just another form of play to children. Children love to turn around and around until they get dizzy and fall down. The ground is not a scary place to children. Falling down and rolling around on the ground are wonderful things for kids to do.

Now we are all grown up and no longer permitted to play. As we enter adulthood, we usually decide that we must work because we need the money. And we must work out because we want to stay in shape. Notice the use of the four-letter words *must* and *work* in both of those sentences. Somewhere between childhood and adulthood, our play turned into exercise, and our fun was replaced by work. This is problematic. It causes two things to happen. First, most people don't want to exercise because it isn't fun.

Second, we aren't mentally engaged in our physical activity, so we don't get as much out of it as we might.

In addition, if our physical activity isn't fun, then we will look for any excuse to avoid it. Contrast this feeling with playing a game of volleyball, tennis, or baseball. Would you think to yourself, "Do I really have to play?" Or, if you were playing in the pool with your friends would you say, "When will we be finished?" No. In fact, when we are having fun, time goes by rather quickly. We want the moment to last, and we look forward to the next time we will have the opportunity.

When we view our physical practice as work, very often, we will mentally check out. This is why you see so many people watching TV or reading a book while they are running on a treadmill. They just want to get it over with. Or they might be listening to music or an audiobook while running around and around the block. Every movement that we make is a work of magic or art. How does the brain send all the right signals to just the right muscles to contract just hard enough at exactly the right time? It is miraculous. Just imagine if you had to consciously control the contractions required by every muscle in your hand just to perform the simple task of picking up a glass of water. It is an overwhelmingly difficult job.

If our exercise is fun, then we will want to do it. Most people run away from activities that are not fun. The brain likes novelty and fun at any age, and it wants to avoid boredom. Do you recall being a child and that your worst fear was that you might be bored? New things are exciting. We need to keep our activities fresh. If we truly want to practice quality movement skills and our practice is fun, then we will be mentally engaged in the task. Positive emotion coupled with intense focus helps quickly create new motor movement patterns in the brain. This is what will make us feel better and move more efficiently.

And isn't one of the things we want to get out of our physical activity the ability to move better? I certainly hope so. Getting better at a physical movement requires that we have a concept or an image of what the desired movement will be. It requires that we execute that movement. And then it requires that we observe the outcome. Did I execute the move as I had envisioned it? Was the timing of all the muscular contractions exactly right? How was my balance? What was the outcome of our efforts? When we are mentally engaged in our physical activity, we will notice how our bodies move. When our minds are somewhere else during our exercise, we will continue to practice any poor or compromised movement patterns, and we won't even notice or care. As a result, we will not get better. We might sweat or breath hard, but our skills will be unlikely to improve.

The structure and function of the human brain are a direct result of the stimulus received. We adapt to our environment during infancy and adolescence. Yes, this adaptation continues throughout our lives; however, the process of modeling the brain is much more pronounced in the early years of life. In this stage of life, we can much more easily form the neural connections required by our external world. In his book, *Play*, Dr. Stuart Brown says, "Play seems to be one of the most advanced methods nature has invented to allow a complex brain to create itself."[21] Notice that he says "create itself." Our brains must be molded to fit our environments. When we are born, we have essentially a blank slate. What language will I need to speak? What is the terrain around me that I must master for hunting? Our parents, those around us, and the world

---

[21] Stuart Brown, *Play: How It Shapes the Brain, Opens the Imagination, and Invigorates the Soul*, With Christopher Vaughan (New York, Penguin Group, 2009), 40.

in which we must survive create much of the way our brain works.

For the first few years of our lives, the only thing we care about is play. But play, in humans, does not end when we reach adulthood. Our daily lives are not completely filled with eating, sleeping, working, and avoiding danger. We have ample time for play, and we need this in our lives. We seek out art, music, sports, movies, card games, social interactions, and the like. We must have play. Why is this? We must play because it stimulates the brain in novel and varied ways that other real-life activities cannot.

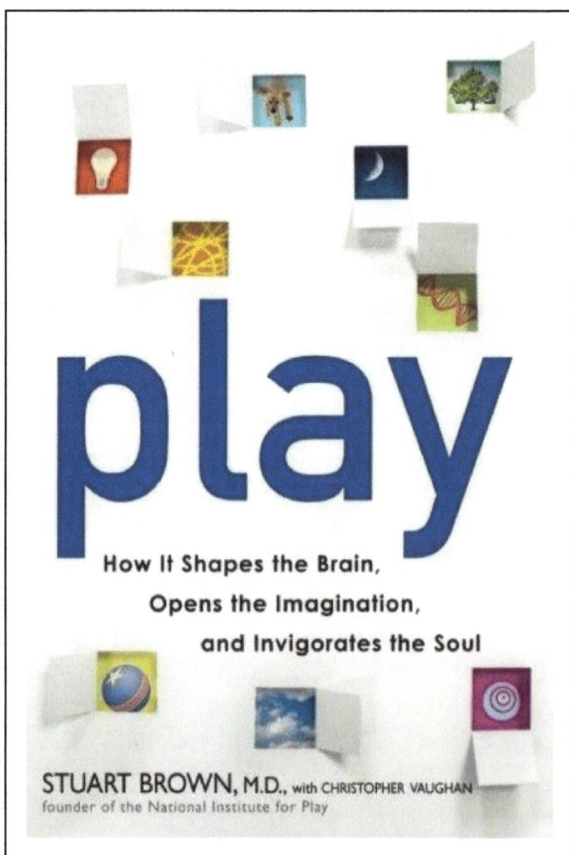

play

How It Shapes the Brain,

Opens the Imagination,

and Invigorates the Soul

STUART BROWN, M.D., with CHRISTOPHER VAUGHAN
founder of the National Institute for Play

Children start life with limited movement skills. First they learn to roll over, then they learn to sit, then they begin to crawl, and soon they are walking. Each of these movement skills is essential to high-quality athleticism later in life. If toddlers walk too soon and don't spend enough time practicing their crawling skills, then they may miss out on some essential development. This can cause compensations in other movement patterns as they mature. In order to improve some desired athletic movement skill later in life, they may need to return to this crawling pattern and practice it.

> *Practicing basic movement patterns such as crawling can often improve other athletic skills.*

Once we begin to stand up, walk about, and say a few words, the adults around us immediately tell us to sit down and shut up. This is strange. We have a lifetime to be serious and to learn mathematics and philosophy. However, we only have a short period in our lives during which we can freely play, learn how our bodies move, and find out how to interact with the world and people around us. The movement skills that we learn during this period are essential to our ability to move well as we mature. As toddlers and children, we must run, jump, roll over, fall down, turn around, climb, and swing. It will also improve our athletic abilities if we spend time hitting, throwing, kicking, and swimming. All these activities encourage our muscles and bones to develop athletically and our nervous system to connect the brain to the body as well as to provide stimulation to our visual and vestibular systems.

Because play causes us to be more "in the moment" and because it is a fun, positive emotional experience, play is the ideal way to improve our talents as an adult. I know that we must be absolutely serious and approach our training and exercise as though they are work. However, work, exercise, and training all often have negative connotations of things that we must do even if we don't want to. But we are less likely to do those things that we don't want to do, and we are likely to do them for a shorter period of time. What if you couldn't wait until the next time you had the opportunity to train? What if you thought about your next practice often throughout the day and looked forward to it with anticipation? Perhaps you would spend time visualizing the perfection of your skill. If you enjoy your training, then you will be in a better emotional state, your practice will be more productive, and you will build myelin faster. In short, you will more quickly develop or improve your desired skill.

Paradigm Shift

Have you ever noticed that when you are sick, under a lot of stress, or fatigued, you perform poorly — you are weaker, you have poor balance, and your vision is not as good as it usually is? These are all indicators that the brain is in charge. Your athletic capabilities are changing from day to day and moment to moment.

The brain is accepting a huge amount of sensory input, processing it, and based on that processing, it is deciding how well it will let you perform. Yes, your conscious brain can sometimes override some of these things. This is what focus and willpower do. But there is much more going on in the brain's processing that is outside the reach of our conscious abilities.

If you have been exposed to the "magic" of brain-based training, then you know what I am talking about. A vision drill, a piece of tape, or a joint exercise has the ability, if it is something that makes your brain happy, to significantly improve your strength or to eliminate pain.

Here is one event that helped cement this concept and encourage me to make a paradigm shift. I was at a Z-Health workshop, and we were looking at neural pathways. One of the trainers there asked me what movement skill I would like to improve. I have been working on my flexibility, specifically a variety of splits, for a couple of decades. You may have no desire to do the splits, and this skill is largely unnecessary for quality athletic performance. However, I am a Tae Kwon Do practitioner. One of our specialties is the execution of kicks to the head, and this requires some flexibility. Somehow, I translated that into a need to do the splits, and I have been somewhat obsessed with this ability

One version of the splits that had eluded me is called the *straddle splits*. I showed my trainer an attempt at this flexibility demonstration, and I was not very close to reaching the floor. The short version of this story is that he put a small piece of tape on my back, and I was immediately able to drop into the full splits. We took a photo and posted it on my Facebook page.

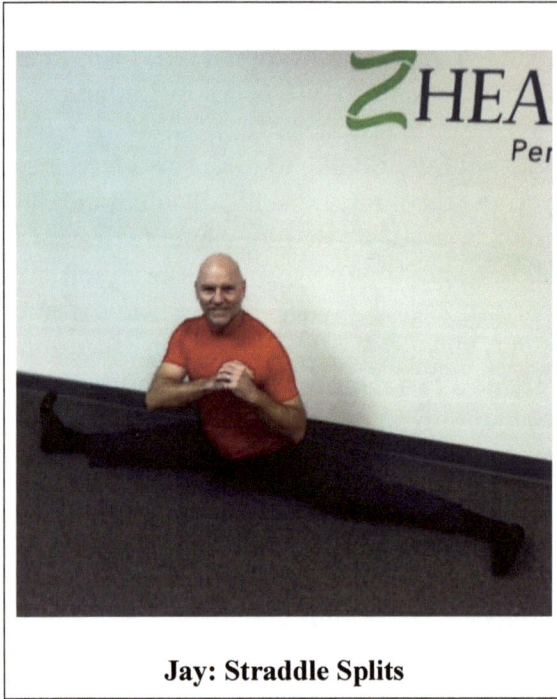

Jay: Straddle Splits

What I now understand is that the brain is in charge. *Any* appropriate change or stimulus to our sensory inputs can have a positive impact on our central nervous system. When the brain wants to, it can increase our strength, improve our balance, or give us more flexibility. Anything can cause anything. This is neither good nor bad. It simply is. If you drink too much, are under a lot of stress, or haven't been sleeping well, then your performance will probably suffer, you might have pain, or your muscles may be weak. Conversely, if you once again begin to use muscles or joints that have been underutilized for a long time, then the sensory input may wake up parts of your brain and help you reach new levels of athletic performance or eliminate chronic pain. And this can happen instantaneously.

Chapter 4: Sensory Inputs

The brain or the central nervous system is in charge of virtually everything in our brain/body system. The brain's primary objectives are survival, movement, and prediction. It is constantly receiving data from the body and the outside environment and using this information to carry out its objectives. Most of the sensory input is not processed on a cognitive level, since this amount of information would prove to be too much for us. We can only direct our focus on a few things at a time like the text message we just received, the mosquito that is buzzing about us, or the red light up ahead. But we can turn our attention to specific sensory inputs if we want to. This is, in fact, how we will go about making changes and improving the brain/body system—through focused or deep-quality practice.

What is happening with all the rest of the sensory input data that is constantly bombarding the central nervous system? It is all being processed, but much of this information is used for comparison with anticipated or expected inputs. Only if we feel, see, or smell something unexpected, novel, or unusual does this new sight, sound, or feeling receive any special attention.

Here is an example. You reach for a bottle of water, remove the cap, and take a drink. This is a surprisingly complex sequence of actions and movements. Yet you probably won't consciously think about it unless…Suppose you cannot get the cap off. What if the water has a funny taste because it has been sitting in your hot car for a month? Will you notice if you spill some of the water because you missed your mouth?

Much of what we see, feel, smell, and taste goes unnoticed because everything is exactly as it should be, exactly as it has always been, and it does not present us with any novel or threatening stimulus. Since we want to cause the brain/body system to undergo positive adaptation and to improve some skill, we will be looking for novel stimuli so that the brain will notice. Let's look at some of the types of sensory inputs that the central nervous system must deal with on a continuous basis.

Joints and Proprioception

Today's increasingly popular *movement training* programs are specifically focused on joint mobility exercises. Move the feet, ankles, knees, hips, and so on. Move all the joints in the body back and forth and in circles while making sure to use every joint. We are looking to improve the way we move; therefore, a lot of our practice will center on the movement of our joints. But there is certainly much, much more information we can use to stimulate the central nervous system, thereby causing positive changes in the brain. The brain will then respond by making us more athletic and by causing physiological adaptation and improvement.

The brain receives sensory information from all parts of our body, including our vision, vestibular system, skin sensations, feelings in our belly, and so on. A significant amount of this sensory information comes from our joints via nerve endings called *mechanoreceptors*. The joints are constantly providing feedback so that we know how much pressure is being applied via muscle activation and so that we can identify the current position of each joint. This is one way we understand where we are and where our limbs are in space. As a result of this sensory input and the sensory inputs from our muscles, we hopefully know if our elbow is locked, fully flexed, or somewhere in between.

While this might seem like a minor thing, it certainly is not. Imagine, for example, that you are throwing a punch with your right arm. You begin with your fist near your shoulder, turn your hips, and extend your arm, throwing your fist outward toward the target. One thing that happens in this movement is that your triceps, the muscle group on the back side of your upper arm, contract in order to straighten your elbow joint. And straightening or extending your elbow is an essential part of throwing a punch. However, if left unchecked, the rapid contraction of the triceps muscle group can easily hyperextend the elbow. This will cause pain and possibly some damage to the elbow joint. To prevent this from happening, the biceps muscle group on the front side of the upper arm contracts as the elbow nears the fully extended position. This acts as "brakes," and those brakes are applied to protect you. How soon are the brakes applied, and with how much force are they applied? This depends on your training and on the brain's awareness of the position of the elbow joint. The more clearly the central nervous system can sense and predict the positioning of the elbow joint, the later during the punch the brakes can be applied. This means that with sufficient, diligent practice, you can learn to punch harder and faster. This means that you will become a more efficient athlete. You will be quicker, and you will not be fighting against your own muscular tension.

This type of training applies to all our joints. The central nervous system uses the sensory input from all our joints to enable us to perform quality, efficient athletic movements. There is a high concentration of sensory neurons located within our joints. But much of this information is processed outside our consciousness. To become better athletes, we must rewire our nervous system so that we have high-quality, fast, and clear communication between the brain and our body parts. And this information must be as accurate as possible. This will require training for most of us. If we can precisely sense how our joints are positioned, then we can move more quickly, with more force, and with improved timing. In short, we will be better athletes.

Conversely, we can have poor sensory information regarding the position of our joints. This reduced proprioceptive feedback will not allow the brain to efficiently control our bodies' movements. We will have fuzzy or unclear movement maps in our brain. When the central nervous system doesn't clearly know where a body part is or how to move that body part, it is a threat to our survival. Threats to our survival cause the brain to become unhappy, which can cause it to express this unhappiness to us via pain, weakness, reduced speed of movement, or poor balance.

> *Poor movement quality is a threat to our survival.*

If we have a joint that doesn't move well, then the brain can communicate this to us in one of its many ways. The chronic pain in your shoulder can be the brain's way of telling you that you lack quality movement abilities in your hip. Therefore, it is possible that practicing accurate movements with your hip and improving the associated neural pathways can make your shoulder pain disappear.

We can use our knowledge of skill acquisition to improve our proprioception. When we learn to move any joint with accuracy and control, we are clarifying the movement map and growing new myelin on the neural pathways associated with that movement. Frequent, deep, focused, quality movement practice is the best way to learn to move well.

Walking and Back Force Transmission

When most people think of the body, they visualize a system of bones, muscles, tendons, and ligaments. Perhaps they will think of veins, nerves, and internal organs. This view of the body makes sense, since these are the structures we will see in any anatomy book.

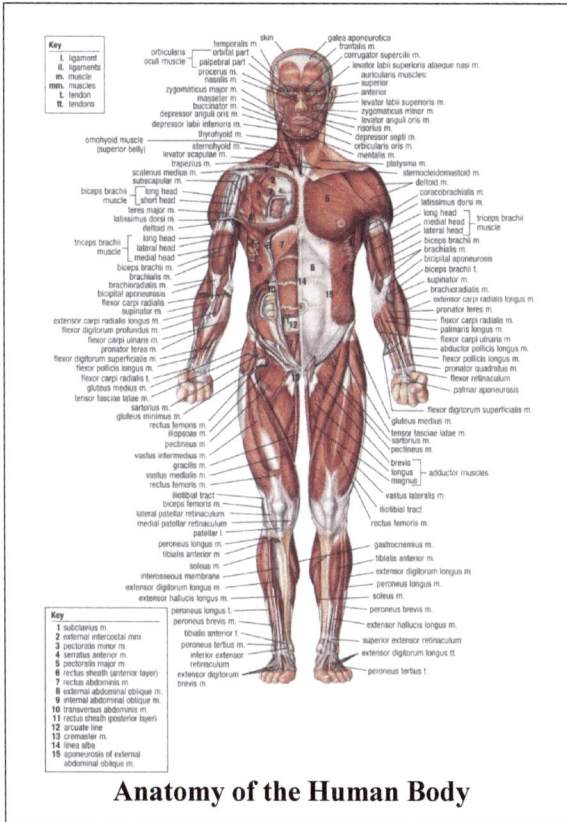

Key
l. ligament
ll. ligaments
m. muscle
mm. muscles
t. tendon
tt. tendons

skin
temporalis m.
orbicularis — orbital part
oculi muscle — palpebral part
procerus m.
nasalis m.
zygomaticus major m.
masseter m.
buccinator m.
depressor anguli oris m.
depressor labii inferioris m.
thyrohyoid m.
omohyoid muscle (superior belly)
sternohyoid m.
levator scapulae m.
trapezius m.
scalenus medius m.
subscapular m.
biceps brachii — long head
muscle — short head
teres major m.
latissimus dorsi m.
deltoid m.
triceps brachii — long head
muscle — lateral head
— medial head
biceps brachii m.
brachialis m.
brachioradialis m.
bicipital aponeurosis
flexor carpi radialis
supinator m.
extensor carpi radialis longus m.
flexor digitorum profundus m.
flexor carpi ulnaris m.
pronator teres m.
flexor digitorum superficialis m.
flexor pollicis longus m.
flexor carpi radialis t.
gluteus medius m.
tensor fasciae latae m.
sartorius m.
gluteus minimus m.
rectus femoris m.
iliopsoas m.
pectineus m.
vastus intermedius m.
gracilis m.
vastus medialis m.
rectus femoris m.
iliotibial tract
biceps femoris m.
lateral patellar retinaculum
medial patellar retinaculum
patellar l.
peroneus longus m.
tibialis anterior m.
soleus m.
interosseous membrane
extensor digitorum longus m.
extensor hallucis longus m.
peroneus longus t.
peroneus brevis m.
tibialis anterior t.
peroneus tertius m.
inferior extensor retinaculum
extensor digitorum brevis m.

galea aponeurotica
frontalis m.
corrugator supercilii m.
levator labii superioris alaeque nasi m.
auricularis muscles:
superior
anterior
levator labii superioris m.
zygomaticus minor m.
levator anguli oris m.
nasorius m.
depressor septi m.
orbicularis oris m.
mentalis m.
platysma m.
sternocleidomastoid m.
deltoid m.
coracobrachialis m.
latissimus dorsi m.
long head — triceps brachii
medial head — muscle
lateral head
biceps brachii m.
brachialis m.
bicipital aponeurosis
biceps brachii t.
supinator m.
brachioradialis m.
extensor carpi radialis longus m.
pronator teres m.
flexor carpi radialis m.
palmaris longus m.
flexor carpi ulnaris m.
abductor pollicis longus m.
flexor pollicis longus m.
pronator quadratus m.
flexor retinaculum
palmar aponeurosis
flexor digitorum superficialis m.
gluteus medius m.
tensor fasciae latae m.
sartorius m.
pectineus m.
brevis
longus — adductor muscles
magnus
vastus lateralis m.
iliotibial tract
rectus femoris m.
gastrocnemius m.
tibialis anterior m.
extensor digitorum longus m.
peroneus longus m.
soleus m.
peroneus brevis m.
extensor hallucis longus m.
superior extensor retinaculum
extensor digitorum longus tt.
peroneus tertius t.

Key
1 subclavius m.
2 external intercostal mm.
3 pectoralis minor m.
4 serratus anterior m.
5 pectoralis major m.
6 rectus sheath (anterior layer)
7 rectus abdominis m.
8 external abdominal oblique m.
9 internal abdominal oblique m.
10 transversus abdominis m.
11 rectus sheath (posterior layer)
12 arcuate line
13 cremaster m.
14 linea alba
15 aponeurosis of external abdominal oblique m.

Anatomy of the Human Body

However, surrounding each muscle is a strong, stretchy substance, somewhat like plastic food wrap, called *fascia*. This material permeates our bodies. It is used to hold all the muscles together and is essential so that the muscles can apply force to the bones they move.

Fascia may look like a plastic bag holding all the muscles in place, but it is much more important than that. Fascia is innervated, providing sensory information to the central nervous system, and fascia gives us strength to perform movements with efficiency. How does fascia give us efficient strength?

Picture a Swiss exercise ball, the kind you will find in most gyms. It is made of a stretchy rubber material and filled with air. When you sit on the ball, it compresses, stores some energy, and then it rebounds. You sit on it, you bounce, and you are propelled upward. This is one of the functions of fascia, the storage of energy for later usage. It often acts like a rubber band. When you pull it one way, it elongates and resists the movement. When you let go, it returns to its original position.

Fascia is living material and is subject to the same rules of adaptation. It is constantly changing as a result of the movement you do and the forces applied to the tissue. In fact, this body structure adapts quite quickly. Strong, active people have strong fascia. In fact, when you see someone who appears wiry or sinewy, much of this appearance is due to thick, strong fascia. This is why wild game is tough and chewy. Animals in the wild are more athletic, if you will. Domesticated animals have comparatively less fascia, and their tendons and ligaments are not as strong. Their tissue has less rubbery coating, and so the meat is much more tender. (Cows don't move much, and their meat would still be quite tender if they watched television and spent time on social media with other cows.)

As we discussed earlier, if you are like most people, then the most important exercise you are doing to cause adaptive changes to your body and brain is walking. You perform thousands of repetitions of this exercise each day. Because our brain/body system wants to be efficient, walking makes extensive use of our fascia.

Imagine a photo is taken of you while you are walking. In this hypothetical photo, you are taking a step with your left leg forward and your right arm forward. The fascia running from your right arm across your back to your left leg stores energy in an elastic system we will call a *sling*. You can think of this like the act of stretching a rubber band. The band stores some energy and then it wants to return to its original position. This act of returning to its original shape does not require additional energy from us. The contracting fascia helps pull our right arm and our left leg backward so we easily move forward. There are many of these facial sling systems in our body so that we use less energy when performing athletic movements.

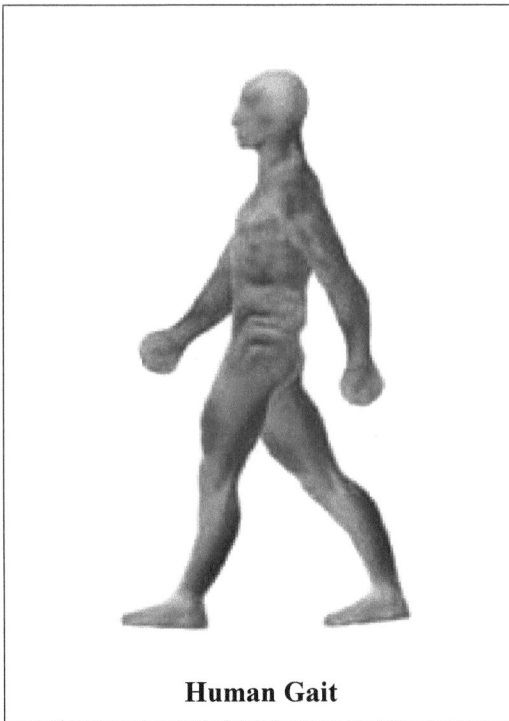

Human Gait

After your right arm is forward and your left foot is forward, you will complete the step. Then your left arm will be forward and your right foot will be forward. As you can see, there are two sling systems crossing on the back side of your body. We will call these two sling systems the *back force transmission system*.

There is also a pair of slings on the front side of the body. Returning to our original photo where your left leg was forward and your right arm was forward, let's look at the other limbs. Your left arm is back, and your right leg is back. This causes a stretch from the left arm across the front of the body and down the front of the right leg. You have two slings storing energy on the front of the body. The two sling systems on the back are designed to be balanced, as are the two sling systems on the front. When these sling systems are not in balance, some additional and therefore inefficient energy must be applied from our muscles to help us walk, stay upright, and stay in balance.

Although Thomas Myers's book can be a bit technical, *Anatomy Trains* is an excellent treatise on the way that fascial slings, or myofascial slings, work in the human body.[22]

---

[22] Thomas W. Myers, *Anatomy Trains: Myofascial Meridians for Manual & Movement Therapists*, 3rd ed. (London: Churchill Livingstone, 2014).

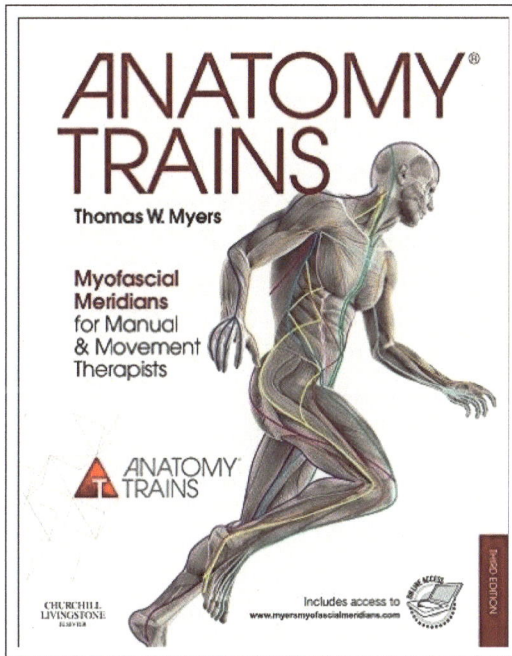

Why are these fascial slings so important? Fascia is one of the first and fastest tissues to begin the structural adaptation process. Fascia thickens and provides additional support and increases our elastic energy storage. Likewise, it can act to restrict our movement. How does the body decide where to strengthen or thicken the fascia? The adaptation is based on our most common movement patterns and load demands. Once again, I am simply saying that we are constantly adapting to the movements that we are doing every day. If your movement patterns are inefficient, then you will grow new tissue to support those unathletic patterns.

Another thing of interest here is that our fascia is innervated. This means that the brain is aware of the stresses that are being applied to it. Suppose, for example, that you are a right-handed golfer or a bowler and that thousands of times you have twisted your body from right to left in a counterclockwise direction in order to either throw a bowling ball or swing a club. However, there have not been an equal number of loaded repetitions twisting your body from left to right. What would be a probable outcome of this behavior? The fascia would adapt to support this movement. You will become more efficient at rotation from right to left, or counterclockwise. You will get better at storing energy so that you can execute your desired athletic movements. You will become more proficient at turning from right to left. Your fascia is now out of balance and is compromising your gait (or the way you walk) because your slings have changed. Is it possible that the brain, aware that you are now twisted slightly to the left, can become unhappy about your compromised walking ability? Yes, it could. If you are twisted to your left, then it is unlikely that your gait pattern is as efficient as it could be. Is it possible that you could develop chronic lower back pain because your new skills are interfering with some essential survival skills? Yes, it is possible.

The takeaway here is that fascia exists throughout your entire body. This fascia is highly innervated and adaptive. The fascial structures are constantly changing, and the fascia is reporting information to your brain via sensory input. If your movement patterns are not efficient, then you will adapt, and the brain will know about it.

> *Sensory input from your body's fascia allows the brain to know about your movement patterns.*

Is it possible that your movement patterns have caused changes in your fascia—that you are now tight or restricted in what used to be normal athletic movements? Could this restriction cause the brain to know that your movements are compromised? Yes, this is likely. When the brain becomes aware that you have lost some movement skill that is essential for your survival, it will try to communicate this unhappiness to you. Could a simple, repetitive movement (like using a mouse or carrying a purse) cause a pain or reduced function in some other part of your body? Yes, this is possible.

Respiration

Breathing is important. Just hold your breath for five minutes while you meditate on this subject and soon you will, no doubt, agree with me.

Recognizing that breathing is important is a simple but rather profound realization that can begin changing most people's paradigms. Why? Because, unfortunately, we take breathing for granted. If I told you I could help you breathe better, then wouldn't you likely think, "That's silly. I already know how to breathe"? If things are going well, then we mostly breathe without conscious thought. Our respiration is the result of years of habit. And we believe we are rather good at it.

Respiration does some important things for our bodies. Our lungs remove the carbon dioxide from our body and replenish our blood with oxygen. This blood gas exchange process also helps control the pH of our blood. And for proper health, the pH, or acidity, of our blood must be maintained within a very narrow range of acceptable values.[23] Proper breathing also causes the diaphragm muscle, a dome-shaped muscle attached to the bottom of the lungs, to move upward and downward. This action massages our internal organs, helping to ensure their

---

[23] Acceptable human pH levels fall between 7.35 and 7.45. Gerry K. Schwalfenberg, "The Alkaline Diet: Is There Evidence That an Alkaline pH Diet Benefits Health?" *Journal of Environmental and Public Health* Volume 2012 (2012), Article ID 727630, http://dx.doi.org/10.1155/2012/727630.

health. The brain is aware of all these activities or the lack thereof.

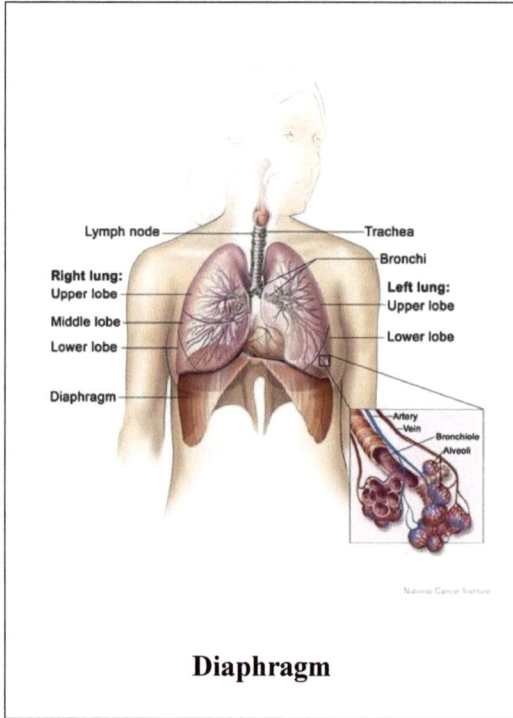

Diaphragm

Breathing is a movement skill, and the brain receives lots of sensory input from this activity. Each inhalation requires the activation of muscles to pull the air into the lungs. Similarly, if we perform a forced exhalation, for example, the act of blowing up a balloon, then we will contract some muscles to force the air out. If we are performing this movement skill efficiently, then our rib cage will expand with each inhalation. If we are to be efficient athletes, then the rib cage should be mobile and free to move up and down and to expand and contract with ease.

We are, unfortunately, spending numerous hours each day sitting at a computer workstation or driving a car. In this seated position, our shoulders are rounded forward and our rib cage is collapsed. This makes proper breathing an impossibility. We simply cannot pull our diaphragm downward because our guts are squished in the seated position. Therefore, we must lift our clavicle and upper chest so that we can inhale. When we do this, the air that we take in does not reach deeply into our lungs. We are using only the upper part of our lungs, and we are practicing a poor movement skill. What happens when we stand up after hours of practicing this inefficient breathing pattern? We continue to "chest breathe" and use the upper portion of the lungs. We no longer use our diaphragm as the primary muscle for our respiration. We no longer expand and contract our rib cage during each breathing cycle. Our organs are not receiving the benefits associated with the massaging motion of proper diaphragmatic breathing.

Each of the twelve thoracic vertebrae in the middle of your spine has a rib attached to it. What happens when the rib cage doesn't move on a regular basis? It adapts and becomes more rigid and increasingly difficult to move. When the ribs become more inflexible, the attached vertebrae no longer move as easily as they should. Let's do a quick count of the vertebrae in our spine. There are seven *cervical* vertebrae for moving the head and neck. There are five large *lumbar* vertebrae in the lower back. And there are twelve *thoracic* vertebrae attached to your ribs. This is half of the bones in your spine! This means that if your rib cage is not mobile because you are not breathing well, then you will seriously compromise the ability of your spine to move into the bending and twisting positions required of an exceptional athlete.

The respiratory system is concerned with bringing in oxygen for the blood and muscle tissues and with expelling carbon dioxide. Oxygen is used to combine with fuel and to produce the energy we need for all bodily processes. Carbon dioxide is produced as a by-product when we use our muscles during any movement. Carbon dioxide drives our reflex to take another breath. It is not that we need more oxygen but that we feel the need to get rid of the carbon dioxide in our bloodstream.

In his book *Close Your Mouth*, Patrick McKeown says that most people breathe too much.[24] We constantly breathe high into the lungs and, as a result, we take too many breaths. Similar to overeating, McKeown says that overbreathing is a habit that leads to many ailments, including asthma. He also claims that overbreathing reduces our carbon dioxide levels too far. We need carbon dioxide to transport oxygen throughout the body. McKeown says:

> *Breathing a volume greater than normal does not improve the amount of oxygen in your blood…instead it lowers CO_2 levels, firstly in your lung, then in your blood, tissues and cells. The greater the amount of air taken into your body, the less oxygen is delivered.*[25]

---

[24] Patrick McKeown, *Close Your Mouth: Buteyko Breathing Clinic Self Help Manual* (County Galway, Ireland: Buteyko Books, 2004).
[25] Ibid., 10.

Close Your Mouth

Buteyko Breathing Clinic self help manual

Stop Asthma, Hay Fever
and Nasal Congestion
Permanently

Patrick McKeown

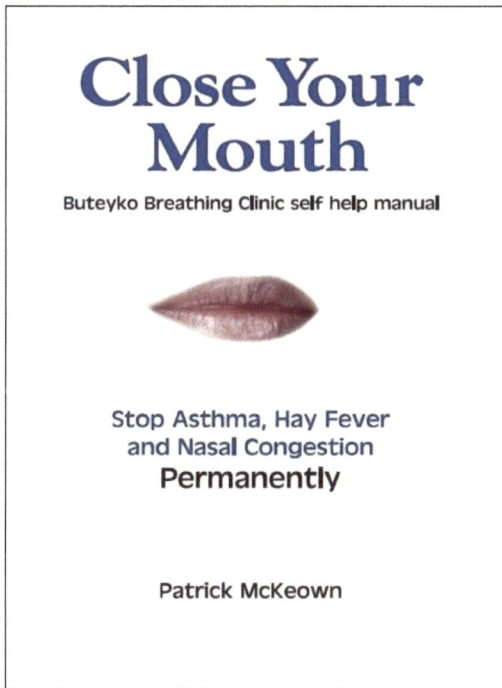

Utilizing the Buteyko breathing method and its training regimen outlined in *Close Your Mouth*, McKeown claims to be able to reduce the symptoms of or cure asthma. Could you learn to breathe better? Yes. This book actually provides a step-by-step method on how to do this.

> *Breathing is essential to our survival; therefore, the brain will complain if our breathing skill is poor.*

The brain's primary objective is to ensure our survival, and breathing is certainly essential for that. Therefore, the brain will become quite unhappy as the quality of our breathing declines year after year. Your spinal mobility will become more restricted, and the ability of your lungs to control your blood pH can be compromised. Conversely, doing a small amount of work to improve the efficiency of our respiratory system can quickly improve your athletic performance or reduce chronic pain. Why? Because having a well-functioning respiratory system will make the brain happy, and it will reward you with increased strength and better stamina.

The Inner Ear and the Vestibular System

Just behind your eardrum lies the seemingly magical vestibular system. This is yet another sensory input system that you might have been taking for granted.

Your eardrum and inner ear are responsible for processing sound. Hearing is an important early warning system. We rely on sound to know more about what is happening in the world around us and to help us sense danger. Therefore, the ability to hear well is very important to the health of the brain/body system. But our ears are not only useful for the enjoyment of music and conversing with our friends.

Here we will talk about the vestibular system, the fast and powerful sensory organs that tell us which way is up and where we are going. This system is a very important part of the sense we call *balance*. Visual and proprioceptive inputs are certainly important for our sense of balance, but if our vestibular system is not functioning well, then we will be unstable. Confusing or mismatched signals from our vestibular system can make us dizzy or nauseous. This is what happens in carsickness. Your eyes say the world around you is stationary because you are not moving relative to the inside of the car. However, your vestibular system is telling you that you are moving—stopping, starting, and turning.

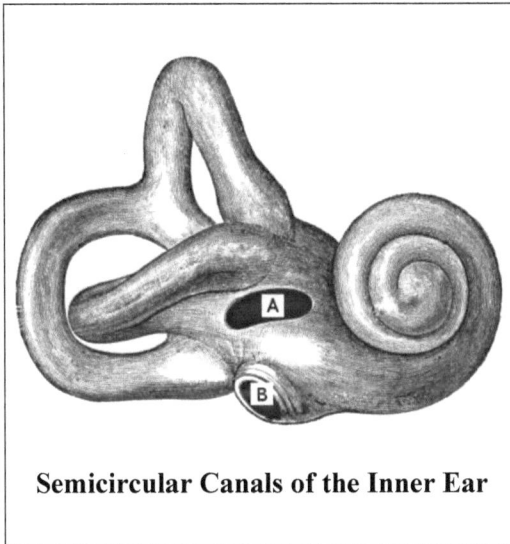

Semicircular Canals of the Inner Ear

In the inner ears are your semicircular canals. Each ear contains three of these canals for a total of six canals. Each canal is filed with a fluid and is lined with small hairs called *cilia*. As you move, the fluid sloshes around inside the canals, pushing on the small hairs. When this happens, the electrical signals being sent to your brain change, thereby indicating that you are changing directions or moving.

There is a large amount of information coming from the inner ear, and this information must be processed quickly and accurately. Here are two important reasons why this system must function quickly: your vision and your postural stability. Let's look at how these systems are supposed to work.

It amazes me that we can walk or ride in a car on a bumpy road and, while doing this, read a book. Our heads are shaking about and the book is unsteady, yet our eyes instantaneously and continuously make all the minute adjustments necessary to keep the image steady. In the early days of video recording, the operator had to take great care to hold the camera steady. If not, then the image would be shaky and unsteady, and these movies would be very irritating to watch. Of course, today, we have image stabilization on our high-tech cameras and even on our smartphones. This image stabilization feature is similar to one of the functions that the semicircular canals perform in concert with the movement of our eyes.

Imagine what happens if the semicircular canals are not functioning as well as they should be. The automatic compensatory movements of the eyes will not occur as accurately or as quickly as they should. We will experience jumpy images of the world around us, and we will no longer want to move. We might feel slightly nauseous or tense and irritated. We might no longer want to move. We need a well-functioning vestibular system in order to keep our athletic vision system working properly.

The semicircular canals are also responsible for the almost instantaneous and seemingly imperceptible corrections to our posture. Imagine you are standing in line waiting for a bus, train, or taxi, and someone in a hurry bumps into you. What happens? Did you fall down? Well, hopefully not. No, your center of balance was disturbed, and the inner ear sensed movement. Immediately, all the muscles in your body went to work to make the necessary minute corrections to your posture. If the vestibular system is not functioning properly, then you will not move well. You will develop an increased and possibly subconscious fear of falling, since this postural control mechanism has been compromised. You might walk around with an overall increase in tension in preparation for your next fall. Or you might walk with your eyes always focused on your feet or the ground immediately in front of you. This is not the way an athlete moves.

The vestibular system is another one of your sensory input systems, and it is very important. How do we maintain proper function of this system? We must use it. When we were children, we loved to play on a merry-go-round and spend time on a swing. We would even turn around and around and around until we got dizzy and fell laughing to the ground. All these activities provided a lot of stimulus to the vestibular system. This also happens when we throw toddlers into the air or bounce them on our knees. We are providing them with much-needed vestibular stimulus.

Now that we are all grown up, what stimulus is our vestibular system receiving? Not much. All day, every day, we are sitting in front of a computer. When we exercise, most activities are either done sitting, lying, or standing, but very little, if any, training involves getting up and down, turning around, or being shaken up. Even most of our "cardio" exercise is performed in a straight-ahead manner that doesn't cause us to turn our heads. How much do we turn our bodies and our heads when we are on a treadmill, a stationary bike, or an elliptical trainer? Even running, which shakes us up a little, is usually performed in a straight line on a smooth surface. We need to move our heads and our bodies in a wide variety of directions to provide adequate stimulus to the vestibular system.

This is one of the great benefits to playing sports. Tennis or racquetball requires you to run around and chase a ball and to react to the flight of the ball. Martial arts practice and dance require you to move in three-dimensional space and to turn around frequently. Team sports such as basketball, soccer, and football require you to move in all directions and to react to the movements of others or to a ball on the field. All these activities provide the brain with much-needed sensory stimulus. These types of activities keep the sensory apparatus of the inner ear functioning and ensure that the central nervous system continues to know how to process this incoming information. If we want our brain to function well, then we must challenge it on a regular basis. The *New England Journal of Medicine* published a study that showed regular dancing and other challenging leisure activities produced a significant reduction in the occurrence and symptoms of dementia and Alzheimer's disease.[26]

Vision

We have talked about the sensory input from our skin, muscles, and joints. This is called *proprioception,* and it gives the brain information about where our body parts are in space. This is how we are able to touch our nose with our fingertip when our eyes are closed. We have also examined the vestibular system located in our inner ear. This is the sensory input system that tells the brain where we are going and which way is up, and it helps control our posture.

The system we are going to look at now is the visual system. Of the three, this system provides this largest amount of information to the central nervous system. Let's compare the amount of data of these three systems using current computer concepts.

If we say our proprioception system is like a Word file, then a document might take ten thousand bytes or ten kilobytes of space on our computer. Then we might say our vestibular system is like a high-definition music file. A music file might take ten million bytes or ten megabytes of space. By comparison, a high-resolution video file might take ten billion bytes of ten gigabytes of space on the

---

[26] Joe Verghese, Richard B. Lipton, Mindy J. Katz, Charles B. Hall, Carl A. Derby, Gail Kuslansky, Anne F. Ambrose, Martin Sliwinski, and Herman Buschke, "Leisure Activities and the Risk of Dementia in the Elderly," *The New England Journal of Medicine* 348 (2003): 2508–16.

computer. Not only do these video files take up more space but also require thousands of times more processing power for your computer to work with them.

Sensory System	Type of File	Size of File
Proprioception	Word Document	10 kilobytes
Vestibular	Music	10 megabytes
Vision	Movie/Video	10 gigabytes

According to some estimates, as much as 50 percent of the neurons in your brain are involved in some way in the processing of information coming from your eyes.[27] Have you ever noticed that you close your eyes when the stress from the world around you just gets to be too much to handle? This frees up lots of processing power for the rest of your problems. To your brain, your visual system is the most important sensory input system. You can detect minute movements almost instantaneously. You can judge distances. And if your eyes are doing their job, then you will be readily able to avoid danger, find food, and chase after a prospective, attractive, and supportive mate.

If our visual system is not functioning well, then it will interfere with the brain's ability to predict the world around us. We will not be able to move as well as we should. In this case, our survival is threatened because we cannot see the bad guys coming.

We are getting better and better at the things we practice the most: (1) looking through the windshield of a car and (2) staring at a computer, tablet, or smartphone. Unfortunately, our eyes are designed to do much more

---

[27] "MIT Research—Brain Processing of Visual Information," *MIT News*, December 19, 1996, http://news.mit.edu/1996/visualprocessing.

than this. They are supposed to take in information from the world around us. This means they should be moving in all directions, changing focal length from near to far, and stabilizing on objects of interest. The center of our vision, or foveal vision, is important, but we also rely on our peripheral vision to provide us with an early warning system. We see or sense movement in our peripheral field, and this potentially tells us we should take a look and see what is going on over there. Here are some of the things the eyes are designed to do.

- Track an object as it moves across our field of view.

- Track an object (or converge) as it moves toward us. (This is important for avoiding spears, rocks, and oncoming bicycles.)

- Change our focus from near to far and back again.

- Stabilize our gaze on objects in a variety of directions and at a variety of distances.

- Use our vision in a variety of lighting conditions from dimly lit to bright sunlight.

There is a lot going on here! There are muscles that must be used regularly to maintain the movement skills of the eyes. Look up and left. Look down and right. The six muscles surrounding each eye are responsible for movements such as these. Additional muscles change the focal length so that we can shift our gaze from far to near.

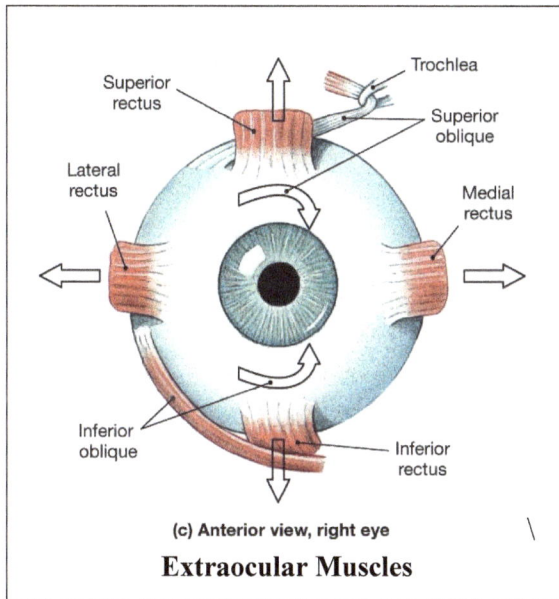

(c) Anterior view, right eye

Extraocular Muscles

Like all skills, eye movement is subject to the use-it-or-lose-it rule. We must maintain the strength in these muscles, and we must have the motor control to accurately position our eyes using these muscles. Then there is the issue of movement. If we cannot accurately and quickly move our eyes, then our athletic performance will be impaired.

Suppose we are throwing or hitting a ball. To perform this skill accurately, we must be able to keep our eyes focused on the ball. However, our head will move as we prepare to throw or hit and will continue moving throughout the action. Therefore, the eyes must move smoothly, quickly, and accurately to counteract the movement of the head. If they cannot do this, then we will not move well or perform athletically. Often, we will find poorly coordinated movement patterns have restricted eye movement or inaccurate tracking as one of their root causes.

As a child, I suffered from myopia, the scientific term for being nearsighted. I didn't even know that I was nearsighted. I always sat in the front row in school so I could see the blackboard. I thought that anyone sitting in the back of the room simply didn't want to learn. Finally, in high school, I was given some glasses to correct my poor vision. Fortunately for me, I didn't start wearing glasses until I was around sixteen years old. Why do I say this is fortunate? Because wearing glasses *will* adversely affect the way we move. "What?" you might ask. Yes, probably all those years of moving and playing without glasses helped me develop better eye movement and better athleticism than I would have acquired had I worn glasses.

Our eyes are supposed to move up, down, left, and right; however, they simply cannot do this when we wear glasses. The center of the lens helps us see things clearly. But surrounding the lens is a frame. We cannot see through the frame, and everything outside the frame is, by nature, unclear. Therefore, we do not move our eyes outside the limits of the frame of the glasses. We also have quite limited peripheral vision for the same reason.

This means that to see something to the left, we cannot move our eyes, but rather, we must move our head or turn our whole body. This is not a very athletic movement pattern, is it? While glasses will definitely help you read the Snellen chart at your optometrist's office, they will not necessarily make you a better athlete. Could your glasses restrict your eye movement, degrade your athletic movement skills, and make the brain unhappy? Yes, it is possible.

E		1	20/200
F **P**		2	20/100
T **O** **Z**		3	20/70
L **P** **E** **D**		4	20/50
P E C F D		5	20/40
E D F C Z P		6	20/30
F E L O P Z D		7	20/25
D E F P O T E C		8	20/20
L E F O D P C T		9	
F D P L T C E O		10	
P E Z O L C F T D		11	

Snellen Chart

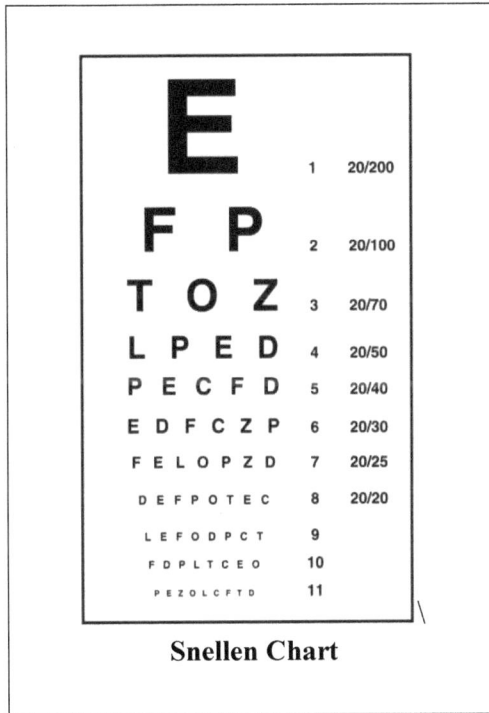

Contact lenses, if you can tolerate them, are a much better solution because they allow normal eye movement. Please remember this statement because we will return to it shortly.

Now, I said that as a child I *suffered* from myopia. This implies that I no longer have this condition. This is correct. I didn't like wearing glasses, and there were numerous television ads that told me I could get laser eye surgery, or LASIK, and my vision would be permanently fixed. (Sort of like getting a brand-new knee.) I thought this was a wonderful idea. I saved up some money and went to see the laser eye doctor. He said that he could fix my vision, but since I was nearing forty years of age, there was a slight problem. After forty, he told me, our ability to see both near and far (also called *focal length accommodation*) becomes compromised. This meant that I could either see far clearly or I could see near clearly but not both. The usual approach is to correct the vision to see clearly in the distance and then to wear "reading" glasses.

I was not too impressed. I had come to see the laser eye guy so that I could stop wearing glasses. Granted, I would only have to wear them while reading, but I would still need glasses. This was not good.

"If it were me," the doctor continued, "I would opt for monovision LASIK eye surgery."

What the heck was this? Laser eye surgery would fix my vision, and no glasses would be required. I was excited and ready to sign up for the program. Well, let me tell you how this actually worked. They used a sharp instrument to cut a flap into the cornea and peel it back. This provided access to the lens of the eye. Then, using a computer-guided laser, they vaporized some of the tissue of the lens, thereby changing its shape. The new, albeit slightly smaller, lens now focused as desired. This is the short version of what LASIK eye surgery was like when I had it done.

But what is monovision surgery? This is when they repair one eye so that it sees clearly at a distance and they modify the other eye so that it sees clearly up close. When the laser eye doctor/salesman told me about this I asked, "How will the brain know which eye to use?" He told me that the brain would ignore the other eye, the one that didn't focus properly. He said it would take a week or so to get used to it. Of course, I trusted the doctor. Doctors have extensive education and always have our best interests at heart.

The surgery was a success. After the procedure, I could see very well with my right eye (my dominant eye) at a distance and could read well with my left (nondominant) eye. So, what am I complaining about? It's simple, really—you have two eyes for a reason.

If you have normal vision, then the information from each of your eyes is slightly different. This is good because the two images are compared in order to give you a three-dimensional perception of the world around you. However, if the image from your left eye is dramatically different from the other eye's image, then the brain will have trouble resolving the discrepancy. You will always be slightly disoriented as a result of this confusing sensory input.

With only one eye, your vision is two dimensional and lacks the ability to perceive depth or how far an object is from you. This is a clear threat to the central nervous system. When a pinecone, rock, or spear is flying at you, it is rather important that you be able to judge how far away the object is and how fast it is approaching. This will allow you to take evasive action. As if you needed another reason, another way that monovision interferes with your natural athletic ability is that somewhere between *far* and *near* your brain must switch between the two eyes. Far away, I would use my right eye. Up close, I would use my left eye. But as an object, such as the foot of my Tae Kwon Do opponent, approached my face, there would always be a place where the brain was unsure which eye it could count on. Therefore, tracking an object became a problem. And as with most problems of this nature, the brain just compensates. It was unable to tell me that there was a problem. I just felt poorly and began to move less athletically.

What did I do about this? I said we would come back to this. Contact lenses, if you can tolerate them, are a much better solution because they allow normal eye movement. Now I wear one contact lens in my left eye so that the vision from both of my eyes is roughly the same. For really small print, I might need to wear reading glasses, but in general, I don't wear glasses.

The lesson here is that we take our vision for granted. Glasses and eye lens-vaporizing surgery are examples of how we fail to see (no pun intended) how our eyes must work in order for us to move athletically. Your brain thinks your vision system is the most important sensory input system there is. And if you are like most people, then you never do anything to improve the function of this system. We could make some vision training, such as rapidly changing focal length, stabilizing our gaze, and accurately tracking objects as they move through space, part of our regular practice. Wouldn't it be a good thing if our exercise program actually made us better athletes?

Another brief observation is that the laser eye guy wanted to sell me on the need for surgery on both eyes. One eye already was nearsighted and therefore it saw well up close. Eye surgeons make their living by performing eye surgery. Knee replacement surgeons make money by replacing knees. Could there be a conflict of interest here? Do you really need the recommended surgery?

What Makes Us Better Makes Us Better

When we are ill, we accept the fact that we can be weak, have joint pain, and perform poorly. When we are well again, we expect to once again feel better and move better. But the reality is that anything that makes us better makes the entire brain/body system better. If we are happy and ate well yesterday, then we are more likely to be stronger and have better endurance. Better breathing will make our brains happy, improve our posture, and enhance blood chemistry regulation. Therefore, developing an efficient breathing skill will make us more flexible and improve our balance, even though these seem to be completely unrelated to our breathing skill.

> *When something we do makes the brain/body system better, everything in the brain/body system gets better.*

Sleep is another huge and often overlooked factor in determining how much pain we have and how athletic our movement performance will be. Inadequate sleep and poor-quality sleep will adversely affect our brain's performance, and this can cause us pain, reduce our ability to focus and react, and make us move poorly.

Lack of sleep can put us into an unpleasant cycle. When we don't sleep enough, we perform poorly during the day and must work harder and longer. We might consume more food, more carbohydrates, and more stimulants. These things interfere with our sleep cycle.

More and more people are overweight and are prescribed a CPAP to help them sleep. A CPAP is a device that is strapped to the face to help force air into the lungs. Why do we need help breathing? This is because many people are overweight, they breathe through their mouths, and they do not use their diaphragms properly for respiration. More and more people are looking for sleeping aids, such as prescription drugs, hormones, or herbs, in order to get a full night of restful sleep.

We are designed to use our brains and to move all day. We are also designed to eat nutrient-rich foods when we are hungry and to drink plenty of water to stay hydrated. Then, because we are in balance, when we are tired, we sleep. When this doesn't happen, we will not be the pain-free exceptional athletes we are designed to be.

In this chapter, we looked at a wide variety of sensory inputs that greatly affect the brain: joints and proprioception, fascia, respiration, vision, and the vestibular system. To ensure our survival, improve our movement abilities, and better predict the world around us, all these systems must be performing well. That is why we have them. Whenever one of these systems is functioning at a suboptimal level, the brain will be unhappy, and it will make whatever compensations are necessary to ensure your survival. An unhappy brain will reduce your strength, decrease your range of motion, and interfere with your balance. Conversely, whenever you find a sensory system that is not functioning well and you begin to do the work required to return it to proper function, the brain will be happy, and it will reward you. What will be the form of this reward? Everything will get better. Your chronic pain will decrease or disappear, and your athletic performance will jump to new, higher levels.

Paradigm Shift

Over a period of twenty years of teaching Tae Kwon Do, I developed my own (rather skewed) view, or paradigm, regarding the types of athletes who exist in the world and how they would progress through their years of Tae Kwon Do training. In my mind, I put the incoming students into three categories.

1. Naturally gifted athletes

2. Average athletes

3. Motor morons

In my old paradigm, naturally gifted athletes had better DNA. They would typically pick up the skills necessary for quality Tae Kwon Do performance very quickly. Unfortunately, since they picked up the skills quickly, they also became bored quickly. The progression through the Tae Kwon Do belt system is not a fast one. Therefore, after a few months to a year, they would generally stop attending classes and move on to another interest.

Continuing with this paradigm description, we have average athletes. This is by far the largest percentage of new, incoming students. They move reasonably well but are not exceptional. They may or may not have much strength or flexibility. However, they enjoy the challenge of Tae Kwon Do training and are constantly improving — learning new movement skills and challenging their balance and flexibility. Lifelong practitioners and Tae Kwon Do masters usually come from this group.

Lastly, in my old paradigm, are the motor morons. These students moved poorly, had poor balance, and did not learn new skills well. They might work hard and make some improvement, but the gains were slow. After many years of training, they still did not look like high-level athletes. Tae Kwon Do improved their movement abilities and gave them new confidence, but something was still holding them back.

Here's how my paradigm has changed.

Naturally gifted athletes are people who received appropriate sensory stimulation at the ideal time during their development. This enabled them to create better and clearer sensory and motor maps at an earlier age. Then they were generally exposed to a wide variety of movement skills, play, and sports. By the time I was introduced to them, their vision and vestibular systems worked well, and they had a large repertoire of quality movement skills. With this basis, they were able to learn new skills easily.

On the other end of the spectrum are the motor morons. They did not receive enough sensory stimulation or it was the wrong type or it was at the wrong time. They could have also had a physical problem with their visual or vestibular systems. Then, as a result of this, they were behind in their movement skill development. All this means they didn't want to play and didn't want to be involved in sports. Their skills, as a natural consequence, fell farther behind.

How does this paradigm shift help me be a better coach and trainer?

I now recognize that everyone is unique. The amount and type of sensory stimulation that will help *you* improve is different from that which will help *me* improve. What is too much for the motor morons may be not nearly enough for the gifted athlete. The natural athlete will require more challenge, or he or she will become bored. And we must be careful about how much stimulus we pile onto the motor moron. We can easily overload him or her. It all depends on the individual. We might need to go back to basic childhood movements and relearn those skills. Given just the right type, quantity, and intensity of sensory stimulation, every athlete can make significant performance gains. I now believe we all can, with the right kind of diligent, focused work, become the exceptional athletes we were meant to be.

Chapter 5: What Is Pain?

Most people do not like to experience pain. Yet many people accept that growing old means we are supposed to be in pain, and we should just learn to live with it. I have often heard someone say, "It is hell to get old" or "We all just fall apart with age" or "This is just part of the aging process." But this is untrue. You can be pain free and move well at any age. Yes, we are mortal. But most people are in pain and move poorly far earlier than necessary. I have worked with many clients in their twenties and thirties with serious chronic pain. In most (but not all) cases, the primary cause was poor movement.

Pain exists for a reason. Pain is not a punishment. Pain is a construct of the brain to tell us to change our behavior. In other words, it is an *action signal* from the brain. Your arm has gone to sleep, so you should move it. You find your foot in an ant bed where you are enjoying the numerous expressions of love from the fire ants, so your brain says, "Move, you dummy!" You put your hand into a flame, and your brain quickly tells you to stop doing that. These experiences of pain are necessary. One of the symptoms associated with the disease leprosy is that the victim often cannot feel pain. This also can happen with diabetes, as sensory input from extremities is reduced. The inability to feel pain is dangerous and can be life threatening. We need to know when we are damaging our bodies. So, all pain is not bad. We might want to avoid the feeling associated with ant bites, but if we are standing in an ant bed, then we need to know about it quickly.

Acute Pain

The types of pain just mentioned are acute pain. They are the result of tissue damage such as burns, bites, scratches, cuts, and the like. In all these cases, we can, if we look through a microscope, see cellular damage. Associated with this tissue damage is inevitably swelling (or edema), bleeding, or bruising. Immediately after the tissue damage has been detected, our body begins its miraculous healing process. Many different substances, the inflammatory soup, are dispatched to dispel the bacterial invaders and to begin to repair the damaged tissue. This means that scar tissue will be created to mend the fascia, skin, muscles, and bone.

Usually, but not always, we will be aware of the injury at the time it occurs. Right now, we are very aware that we kicked the foot of the bed with our little toe again. Quite often, there is a pause before the pain appears. Then the pain shows up, and it is quite excruciating. A little while later, we are wondering where the pain went. We can see that we have a cut, scratch, or bruise, but it no longer hurts much.

We might have a big injury, like a gunshot wound, and not even know it. The people next to you might think you lost your hand in the paper shredder when all you experienced was a little bitty paper cut. One of the things we must acknowledge as we begin to change our paradigm is that the amount of pain we experience is not directly related to the amount of tissue damage. A small injury can hurt a lot, and a traumatic injury might have little or no pain. One of the funniest books I ever read happens to be very instructive: *Painful Yarns* by Lorimer Moseley.[28] Dr. Moseley spent some time watching people as they came into the emergency room. He assessed and rated the severity of their injuries and compared this to their "ouch and moan" quotient, the amount of pain they were apparently experiencing. The result is hilarious. Some

---

[28] G. Lorimer Moseley, *Painful Yarns: Metaphors & Stories to Help Understand the Biology of Pain* (Canberra, Australia: Dancing Giraffe Press, 2007).

people with horrific injuries were jumping about and laughing. Other patients with minor injuries were screaming, crying, and begging for morphine. Everyone's pain experience is unique and very real to them. However, the amount of physical destruction or tissue damage is not directly related to the intensity of the pain.

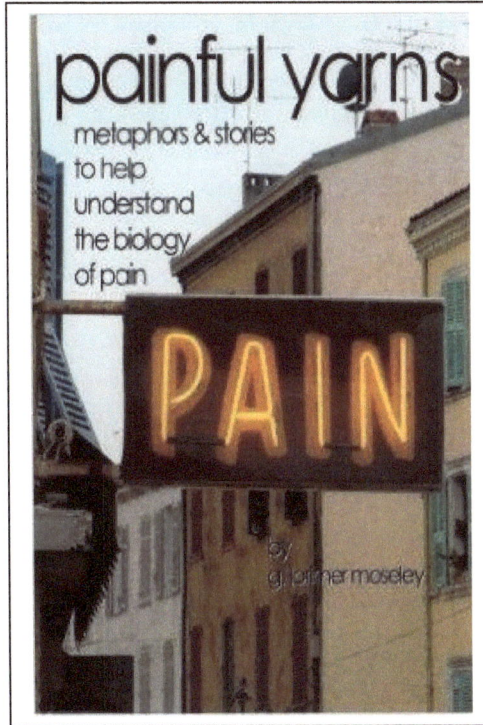

painful yarns
metaphors & stories
to help
understand
the biology
of pain

PAIN

by
g. lorimer moseley

Here is how the damage and repair process (or the injury and healing cycle) normally works. Our bodies are damaged with a cut, scrape, or bruise. Cells are compromised, and we bleed either internally or externally. A flood of inflammatory soup rushes to the site of the wound, causing swelling. The stuff that flows to the place of tissue damage does so to fight off infection, stop the bleeding, and begin the process of bodily reconstruction.

Over the course of a few weeks to a few months, depending on the type of injury, we will undergo a complete healing and remodeling process. In the very beginning, the inflammation process begins to take care of infection. New tissue is grown in excess to repair the tissue. This excess tissue is then discarded, and the scar tissue begins to become softer. At the end of this process, we expect to be healed, recovered, and pain free. That is what is supposed to happen. And we will probably forget about these events unless they are serious and traumatic. (However, I have had clients completely forget about surgeries, broken bones, and gunshot wounds.) We are not designed to remember every scratch, bruise, and skinned knee we ever experienced. Nor are we supposed to have pain after we have healed from those injuries.

For a person with an injury, there is likely no better place on earth to be than America. The American medical system is unsurpassed in fixing your cuts, broken bones, car injuries, and damages caused by disease. If your shoulder is broken, then you can go see a shoulder specialist. If your ear hurts, then you can go see an ear, nose, and throat specialist. We have a specialist for virtually everything.

As children and young adults, we experience lots of (hopefully) minor injuries: cuts, scrapes, burns, and so on. Our brains have become conditioned to associate cause and effect. If we hit our thumb with a hammer, then our thumb will hurt. If we spill hot coffee on our hand, then our hand will hurt. The harder we hit our thumb, the more it will hurt. The hotter the coffee, the greater the damage, and the more pain we can expect. This shapes our paradigm about every pain experience. However, this extensive training that we received early in our lives was mostly about acute pain. We subconsciously believed that all pain, including chronic pain, must be the same and follow identical rules. This is true. All pain follows the same rules. The problem is that we fail to fully recognize and accept the rules of how pain really works. What are the rules? Pain is a creation of the brain, and the central nervous system determines your pain experience based on sensory inputs, history, and emotional context.

Chronic Pain

While we all understand acute pain rather well, there is a different type of pain that is pervasive: chronic pain. Chronic pain is less well understood and rather poorly handled by mainstream Western medicine.

Here is a not-so-fictitious account of chronic pain.

Joe is playing with his son and feels a slight twinge in his right shoulder. Within seconds, the pain disappears. Joe ignores the event. A week later, Joe is working in the backyard and feels the same twinge. This time, it lasts a bit longer. Joe ignores it. Over the next few months, the shoulder begins to ache frequently during the day, but the pain is not severe. Joe ignores it. After a year of this discomfort, Joe begins to take over-the-counter pain relievers (because that is what the commercials say they are for). After all, he is getting older, and everyone his age has aches and pains. Over the next year, the pain continues to increase until Joe, concerned that something is very wrong in his shoulder, goes to see his doctor. After a brief discussion and evaluation, the doctor says he cannot find anything physically wrong with the shoulder. The doctor asks if Joe wants a referral to a shoulder specialist. Joe says no and takes the doctor's prescription for anti-

inflammatory drugs and a stronger pain medication. During the third year, Joe can't take the pain anymore, is convinced he has injured his shoulder, and goes to see a shoulder specialist, an orthopedic surgeon. The surgeon sends Joe for an MRI. The results come back and conclusively show that Joe has a torn labrum and degenerative arthritis in the shoulder. The surgeon recommends that surgery be performed to trim up the labrum and clean up the detritus in the joint. Joe is better after a few weeks. But over the next year, the pain returns, and it is as bad as ever.

Imagine that your shoulder has been hurting for three or four years. Is this an injury that hasn't healed? No. Injuries that don't heal are very dangerous and are probably life threatening. Do you remember the trauma that started this pain? Maybe. Or perhaps not. Even if you remember the trauma, the healing process is the same. The tissue has mended, and the healing process is complete. There should be no pain. Your shoulder is not "injured." The muscles and skin have scarred up, and the bone has been knitted. However, your shoulder still hurts.

If you go see a shoulder specialist, then he or she will likely want to do shoulder surgery to fix the injury. But there is no "injury" because the tissue has healed. It is not really the shoulder specialist's fault. To a hammer, everything looks like a nail. You came to the specialist for a solution to the shoulder problem, and what he or she has to offer are shoulder fixes: pain medication, shoulder rehab exercises, and shoulder surgery. This is how the specialist makes a living. And you want a solution to the pain. The specialist might even do an MRI to "prove" that you have degenerative arthritis in the shoulder that requires this shoulder surgery.

But here is a curious observation. You went to the doctor because your shoulder hurt. The doctor diagnosed you with arthritis and proved it by way of an MRI. But if you had an MRI on the other shoulder, then you would almost certainly find a similar degeneration of the joint structure. In other words, you have arthritis in *both* shoulders. Why does only one shoulder hurt? If arthritis is the cause of the pain, then shouldn't both shoulders hurt?

I have had many clients come to me with chronic pain. They came because they could not resolve their pain issues with mainstream Western medicine. When I took one client's history, I realized this person had had, in two separate cases, more than twenty surgical procedures! In response to this revelation, I incredulously asked, "What kind of doctor would perform this many procedures?" The answer is that the client insisted on these numerous procedures. The client was in pain, and although there was no indication that yet one more procedure would fix the problem, the client didn't know what else to do. And apparently, neither did the surgeon.

Interestingly, *arthritis* simply means pain in the joint. This is from the Latin *arthro* meaning "joint" and *itis* meaning "pain" or "inflammation." You went to the doctor for pain in the shoulder and were diagnosed with arthritis or, in English, "pain in the shoulder"! What did the doctor do for you? Did the doctor give you some pain medications or recommend surgery? Did either of these remedies solve the underlying problem? It is not likely. Unlike bodily trauma and the associated acute pain, the American/Western system of medicine is woefully inadequate when it comes to handling chronic pain. If the pain is not due to an injury, then what is this pain about?

Chronic pain is just like acute pain in that it is a construct of the brain. The brain processes sensory inputs and then decides that this information should be interpreted as a pain event. The input, in this case, is not tissue damage but some other threat. Pain is an experience that the brain provides to tell you that you need to stop doing something, to do something, or to do something differently. In other words, it is an *action signal*. All pain is just that: an action signal.

> *Both acute pain and chronic pain are action signals from the brain.*

The brain wants you to be a fully functional, pain-free athlete. The brain creates pain for a reason: to tell you to do something. Unfortunately, the brain is a poor communicator. It doesn't speak to you in complete sentences and tell you what you need to do to relieve the pain. However, if we learn to listen more effectively, then the brain will tell us what we need to do. Pain is not a random construct. The pain does not appear without reason. If we can find what the brain is telling us we need to do in order to improve our athleticism, then the pain will disappear or will be greatly reduced, and our athleticism will improve.

Pain Is an Action Signal

Part of my paradigm shift is that I now know that diminished athletic performance and chronic pain are different expressions of the same thing. On one end of the spectrum is efficient, tension-free, quality movement, and on the other end is painful, restricted motion. On one end are fast, fluid sport skills, and on the other are weakness and poor balance. If the brain/body system is functioning well, then we will have pain-free flexibility and endurance. If the brain/body system is unhappy, confused, damaged, or inefficient, then we will experience fatigue, weakness, and chronic pain. Chronic pain is an action signal from the brain telling us to stop doing something, to do something differently, or to start doing something that we haven't been doing but that is necessary for our health and survival.

Tissue Damage Does Not Equal Pain

Wouldn't it be great—and simple—if we could tell from the amount of pain we experience exactly how much damage our tissues have incurred? And from our numerous childhood experiences, we usually believe this to be true. But it is not, and we know it is not true. Have you ever been working in the yard or playing with your friends, looked down at your sleeve or pant leg, and noticed that you were bleeding? Did you think to yourself, "What the heck is that? Oh look! I cut myself. I wonder when that happened. Why didn't I feel any pain?" Of course, we immediately ignore this event as an aberration. It is possible to have an injury, even a severe one, and not even notice or have very little pain.

In 2009, a terrorist named Nidal Hasan started shooting people at the Fort Hood army base in my home state of Texas. After the shooting, a young lady, Amber Bahr, applied a tourniquet, made from her blouse, to one of the wounded and was subsequently tending to others. Someone pointed out to her that she was bleeding. She had been shot in the back, and the round had exited her abdomen. She, too, had been wounded in the gunfire but didn't even know it. How can you *not* know that you have been shot? The excitement or fear associated with this horrific event caused her mind to focus on other things, and in determining that these other things were more important than the tissue damage did not create a conscious pain experience.

Conversely, small or even insignificant injuries can evoke an incredible pain response. Just kick the leg of your table with your unexposed toes, and you will probably be disabled for several seconds. Your first thought is "Oh my God! I broke my toe!" Then, you jump around for a bit and rub your toes. Then, just as suddenly as the pain arrived, it disappears. Did the pain disappear because the healing process is complete, and the damage has been repaired? Nope. This intense amount of pain is completely out of line with the injury to your toes. You probably have had similar excessive pain reactions from one of those extremely dangerous lacerations called a paper cut. As you are going through your mail, you tear open an envelope, reach in for this month's electric bill, and *ouch*! You know before you look that it is deep, painful, and will bleed for a long, long time. This might require stitches. You quickly pull back your hand and squeeze on the damaged area, trying to make it bleed. (I don't really know why we do this, except maybe we instinctively want the bleeding process to help clean the wound.) Then, once again, in a matter of seconds, the pain, clearly out of proportion to the emergency-room-necessitating trauma, subsides. And we think, "What the heck is that all about? Why do paper cuts hurt so much?"

From these stories, we know that we cannot trust pain to tell us how much tissue damage we have. Yet we continue to believe that if it hurts a lot, then there *must* be a lot of damage, or the injury must be really bad. This has been a difficult part of my paradigm to try and change. Just because I have a pain in my neck or my knee doesn't mean that I have an injury. And just because it hurts a lot doesn't mean there is a terrible wound. In fact, I probably don't have an injury either big or small. Why? Because you usually know when you damage your body's tissues. You will bleed, it will hurt, it will swell, and you will usually remember when, where, and how you obtained such an injury.

Emotion Influences the Pain Experience

We also tend to believe that pain is an absolute human experience that is consistent from person to person. This means that, for example, if I drop a five-pound weight on my big toe, then it will hurt me the same as dropping a five-pound weight on your big toe will hurt you. But my pain is my pain, and your pain is your pain. For example, we have all seen the differences in reaction to someone receiving an injection. For some little children, it is no big deal. However, even some big, burly men begin to sweat at the thought of a needle and may even pass out as a result of this extremely traumatic experience.

As another example, I frequently put my hands on my clients' ribs above their hips, apply a light pressure, and ask them to inhale and push my hands apart. This encourages them to use their diaphragms to breathe into the lower portion of their lungs. I recently did this to a woman, and she screamed out in obvious agony. She told me that I was squeezing her too hard, crushing her ribs, and she was unable to breath at all. Each of us is clearly unique.

How we think and feel about pain greatly influences our pain experience. Catastrophizing about the pain—"It's getting worse. It's never going to stop! Maybe I'm dying!"—can cause the pain experience to spiral out of control. Yet we can often ignore pain while we are playing and having fun.

For recurring experiences, the pain event can also change as the result of repetition. A pain event can create a memory. And memories become more firmly embedded through repetition. This is like getting better at a skill through diligent, frequent practice. If we view the pain of the injection as bad, horrible, and life threatening, then subsequent injections can become even more painful. If we view the injection as no big deal, then subsequent injections become more routine, less stressful, and less painful. People with a fear of flying, fear of elevators, or fear of heights often increase their fear experiences over time because they are repeating the self-talk that they are afraid, and doom is imminent.

As a martial artist, I have broken hundreds (if not thousands) of boards with my hands and feet. When I break boards, I often see a look of horror or surprise on the faces of those watching. It seems they feel pain because I am hitting or kicking a hard surface. Time after time, I have viewed these breaking events and the slight stinging sensation in my hand or foot as no big deal. Why? To me, it is not painful.

Experience Influences Pain

Pain is a construct of the brain. It is also a subjective experience. The brain is really good at prediction, and as a result, it can create a pain experience based solely on its predictions. Those predictions don't even need to actually happen for the pain to appear.

Recall that most of the input information arriving at the brain is compared to expected results, and then, if all is as it should be, then it is ignored. In other words, most of what we think is happening is due to our predictions. If we perform an action and it causes us pain, then this becomes our prediction. Performing the action many times and experiencing associated pain further reinforces the pain experience. Eventually, due to our practice, we can be sure that this action will cause us pain. In fact, we can become so skilled at generating this pain response that simply *thinking* about performing the action will cause us pain. For this reason, we might not want to practice painful movement. Doing so will simply reinforce the association between the pain and the movement.

> *All quality movement progress begins with one pain-free repetition.*

We can change our pain experience by practicing nonpainful activities. Here is an example of how chronic pain progresses.

One day, Joe notices that his shoulder hurts whenever he raises his arm overhead. Over a period of months, this discomfort continues, and Joe stops attempting to lift his arm overhead because it hurts. When we don't us a body part, we stop receiving sensory input from that movement, and the associated brain maps become cloudy or fuzzy. Over the next few months, Joe learns that his shoulder hurts whenever he raises his arm to eye level. Joe's range of pain-free motion is decreasing. Part of the reason this occurs is that all Joe's experiences with this shoulder are painful. This steady decline in shoulder function combined with increased pain can usually be reversed. The recovery process involves practicing quality pain-free movement. If Joe begins a rehabilitation program that involves challenging the shoulder within the pain-free range of motion, then this action will improve the quality of the brain's maps. This can reduce the threat associated with moving the shoulder. The result will be reduced pain and increased range of motion.

Pain is an interpretation of sensory inputs. Our emotions and memories have an effect on how these inputs are interpreted. When the brain determines that the threat is high enough, one possible outcome is pain. Our prior experiences create memories and directly affect our emotions. Therefore, our experiences can make pain events more intense or, conversely, they can reduce the amount of discomfort we feel.

The Site of Pain Does Not Equal Cause

Another common belief in our paradigm is that if it hurts, then it must be damaged or broken: "If my knee hurts, then there must be something wrong with my knee." This deeply ingrained belief probably comes from the numerous tumbles and falls we had as children. We would trip and bang our knee on the ground. There would be a scrape and associated bruising or bleeding. And yes, there would be pain in the knee. From this, we learned that injury and insult to our knee caused pain, and we made the reverse assumption that pain in the knee meant knee injury. This is not always the case.

Pain is a creation of the brain. Emotion, prior experience, and sensory input are all constantly integrated and interpreted in the brain. This process is continuous and ongoing. If these things predict a sufficient level of threat, then one possible output of the brain is a pain event.

> *He who treats the site of pain is lost.*
> *—Dr. Karel Lewit*

Consider, for example, a condition called *sciatica*. The sciatic nerve is one of the largest nerves in the body. There is one sciatic nerve on each side of your body. It runs from the lower back down each leg, all the way to the foot. Sciatica is caused by compression or irritation of the nerve as it exits the spinal column in the lower back. Sciatica can be very painful. The pain can appear in the hip, the upper leg, the lower leg, and even the foot. But the cause of the pain is an irritation to the nerve in the lower back. There may or may not be any pain in the lower back. The pain can show up virtually anywhere from the top to the bottom of the leg. Now you might be saying, "Yes, but that is different. That is nerve pain." And you would be correct—it is a pain caused by nerve trauma. However, the pain in your foot and your intuition may tell you that you have something wrong with your foot. You might even go to the doctor and say, "There is something wrong with my foot." Hopefully, no one will try to fix your foot. Performing surgery on the foot would not solve the problem because the source of the pain is not in your foot.

Another example involves Head zones. These are areas of the body to which pain is referred when there are problems with our internal organs. In the 1890s, Sir Henry Head discovered that problems in the gut or viscera caused pain to manifest itself somewhere else on the body. Note that this is not a new discovery. One of the reasons the body does this is because we don't have much sensory input or afferent nerves coming from our internal organs. We simply cannot "feel" much pain there. Problems with our pancreas can appear as pain in the lower back or left shoulder. Lung issues often cause pain in the upper back, shoulder, neck, or armpit. Your right shoulder can hurt because of your appendix. And, of course, a heart attack can show up as pain in your left arm. Once again, performing surgery on your left shoulder will not help eliminate your pain if the cause of this pain is your pancreas.

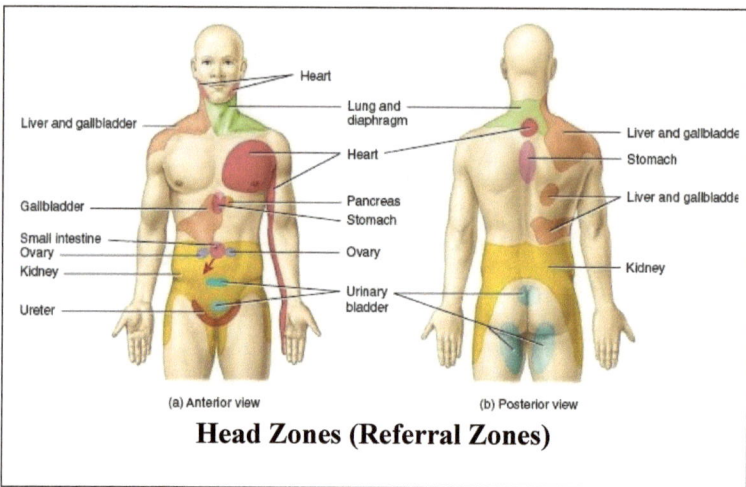

(a) Anterior view　　　　(b) Posterior view

Head Zones (Referral Zones)

Yet we strongly believe that *where* we hurt indicates *what* needs to be fixed. But this is not always the case. This is a difficult change to make in our paradigm.

Have you ever been working in the yard, playing a game, or exercising in the gym when you experienced a sudden, sharp pain somewhere in your body? The answer is probably yes. Then you stopped what you were doing and moved around, and the pain magically disappeared. You thought, "What was that all about?" Then you forgot about it. If this pain was in your hip, for example, then this doesn't mean that you broke your hip. This doesn't mean there is any tissue damage in your hip. This was simply an action signal from the brain. For some reason, the sensory inputs from the body combined with previous experience exceeded some threshold of threat, and the brain responded by creating a pain event.

In our new Z-Health paradigm, we are looking for ways to decrease chronic pain and to improve athletic performance. Often, the pain we are experiencing is simply *not* the result of an injury to that part of the body. Rather, it is a message from the brain that we should do something, stop doing something, or do something differently. In other words, the pain event is an action signal to us from the central nervous system. The action that the brain wants us to take is usually unclear. We must become like Sherlock Holmes and search for whatever will make us better. Reducing the threat will make us better and decrease or eliminate the pain. This is what the brain wants us to do.

Paradigm Shift

In chapter 1, I shared the story of the neck trauma I incurred as the result of high school football. In those days, we were taught to tackle running backs by hitting them in the chest with our heads. We spent lots of time in practice doing exactly this. As you might imagine, this head-smashing practice tends to compress the vertebrae in your neck. Possibly as a result of this activity of my high school years, I subsequently suffered from frequent pain events in my neck. Let's look again at the pain I experienced and what has changed.

Eventually, I became quite frustrated with being unable to move and being in pain, so I went to see the doctor. X-rays showed that I had significant compression and degeneration in my cervical vertebrae. Did I injure my neck? Yes. Probably multiple times on the football field. But those injuries have healed. Because of the condition of the vertebrae in my neck, the orthopedic surgeon recommended that I have some of the vertebrae fused. I refused. As a second choice, the doctors offered me pain medication and muscle relaxers. I did take some of these, but I kept looking for a better solution to my problem. I finally went to see a chiropractor, and this provided some relief.

Standard chiropractic treatment consists of identifying a vertebra that is stuck, immobile, or out of alignment and then adjusting the spine. This adjustment means that the chiropractor holds a vertebra, puts you into a rather scary position, and applies a sudden pressure, causing your spine to go "pop," sort of like cracking your knuckles. The purpose of this process is to mobilize the offending vertebra and to help move it back into proper alignment.

Here is how my paradigm has changed. When I was first introduced to mobility training with a Z-Health, brain-based focus, I learned a series of neck exercises in the R-Phase certification. The purpose of these drills is to maintain or regain the normal movement abilities of the neck. The neck and its vertebrae should be mobile and be able to rotate, glide, and flex.

Within a few months, I completely stopped having painful neck episodes. Why? The pain in my neck was an action signal from my brain. What was it trying to tell me? I had compromised movement in my neck. Remember what the chiropractor was trying to do to my vertebrae? He was trying to mobilize them and put them back into proper alignment. What was I doing? I was avoiding neck movement because I was afraid that it would result in yet another painful neck episode. As a result of my brain-based movement and mobility practice, I was able to improve my neck's mobility.

Perhaps I had a need for an orthopedic surgeon to fuse the vertebrae in my neck. Or perhaps I had a need to improve my own ability to move those vertebrae. As I began to work on neck mobility, the brain became happy. I could move my neck in many ways that I had been avoiding. My pain disappeared. I now know that pain is an action signal. When I have pain, it means I need to change my behavior or exercise routine. My job is to find out what the brain is trying to tell me and to look for what I need to do to make it happy. If I am successful, then the chronic pain will disappear. Now, whenever I have a slight pain in my neck, I immediately go to work. I move my neck a lot! But I only move it in the ways that are pain free. This reminds the brain that my neck does, in fact, move. And it can move without pain.

Chapter 6: Stress and Threat

Your brain is your command center (like the bridge on the starship Enterprise). Data and reports are constantly arriving, and the command center is using this information to decide what needs to be done next. If we see a roaring fire just outside our doorway, then we might make a decision to run away. If we smell food, then we will start to salivate and want to eat. If, however, the sensory input causes the brain to predict that something bad is happening to your body, then the brain can generate some unfortunate outputs. When we are under a sufficient level of threat, the brain will respond by making us weak, reducing our stamina, or causing a pain event. These threats can take many forms: environmental, emotional, imagined, disease, and so on.

Stress Responses

Our brains and bodies are constantly responding to the stresses applied by our environment and from what we do. Hard work applies stress to our bodies, and intense study applies stress to our brains. This is how we improve our physical performance abilities, and this is how we learn new things. So, stress is a good thing, right? That depends on the quantity and type of stresses we are experiencing, how resistant our bodies are to these stresses, and whether we have sufficient time to recover from the damage we sustain.

There are many types of stresses: pollen, pollutants, poor-quality food, lack of sleep, pressure at our jobs, and arguing with our spouses. Regardless of the stressful external or internal stimulus, the brain/body system will generate a response. How do our bodies and brains respond to inputs that they determine are stressful? That depends on how resilient our brain/body systems are and how much more stress we have the ability tolerate at that time.

Exercise is a type of stress. All athletic activity causes wear and tear on the body that must be repaired. This is how we develop stronger muscles and denser bones and improve the function of our nervous systems. We adapt to the challenges of our training. In this case, stress can be a good thing because it makes us better. But this is only true if we are able to tolerate the amount of stress applied. We must have adequate nutrition and enough rest so that we can recover. Then we can potentially become stronger and faster as a result of our practice. If we are run down, eating poorly, or under significant emotional stress, then we may not be able to recover from our exercise activities, and as a result, we might get worse instead of better.

As a personal example, I developed an interest in tearing cards (thanks to a few of my strong friends: Brett Jones, Adam Glass, and Logan Christopher). I asked Logan how I would go about learning to tear a deck of cards. Logan said, "Tear one card, then tear two cards, then…" I have been working on this for a year. So far, the most I have torn is forty-eight cards. But there has been a significant adaptive process to my hands. If I tear too many cards too often, then I can develop an injury and have a setback. Perseverance and persistence are required, but sufficient recovery is also essential. How long will it take for me to be able to tear a full deck of fifty-four cards? It really doesn't matter. I only need to continue trying, learning, and practicing, and I will achieve this goal.

Too much exercise or training without adequate recovery can cause injury to our bones, ligaments, and muscles. Even the function of our internal organs can be compromised. Many endurance athletes such as long-distance cyclists and marathon runners are in nearly constant pain and look quite unhealthy. Young female endurance athletes can suffer from a condition called *athletic amenorrhea,* which causes irregular or cessation of menstrual cycles. Pushing yourself to work harder is admirable in my opinion. I am proud of how I have pushed myself over the years to achieve my goals. However, it is possible to push yourself too hard for too long, and for this, you may pay a high price. We must listen to our bodies.

Many things in our lives can cause us stress. Some of these threats, if intense enough, can evoke the fight-or-flight response. This is what happens when we are in a life-or-death situation. This state of panic begins in the part of the brain called the *amygdala.* As an event such as this unfolds, our heart rate increases, our blood vessels become constricted, our blood pressure increases, and adrenaline is dumped into our bloodstreams. All these things happen in order to prepare us for battle or to escape and help to make us stronger, faster, and better able to survive serious injury. This increase in our abilities happens very quickly. It wouldn't help us to run away from the lion if we are stronger and faster tomorrow. We need it now!

You might think that events that would cause such a radical reaction occur quite rarely. Wild animals do not often attack us, nor are we frequently trying to survive a physical assault by someone wielding a knife. Yet these types of emergency situations are exactly why we evolved our bodies to react this way.

Unfortunately, this intense response often happens to us as an irrational, unnecessary, or unwanted reaction to some daily occurrences. We undergo the very same fight-or-flight response whenever the amygdala turns on in response to a high level of threat. If your spouse expresses extreme displeasure at your behavior, then you might react by turning red. Your breathing may become shallow.

You might feel that you want to run away or break some dishes.

Highly stressful incidents can also occur at your job due to pressure from your boss. As a result, your blood pressure might skyrocket. Being pulled over by a police officer for a traffic violation can make you experience panic. You might begin to perspire. You are not-so-patiently standing in a long line at the grocery store when someone cuts into the line. Your muscles tense, and you get ready to yell at the person. You get the idea. We all too often have these fight-or-flight events. They are not really life threatening, but the physical reaction is identical to the one that occurs when we are chased by a bear.

In our modern, high-stress life, these types of events can occur with disturbing regularity. Whenever we go through one of these high-stress events, the body must clean up the adrenaline that was dumped into the bloodstream. In other words, we must recover. Even though we were not in actual physical danger, our bodies reacted as though our lives were at risk. These emotional events apply a significant stress to the brain/body system. These frequently occurring times when we overreact take a toll on us in the long run.

For an exceptional description of the stress hormone cascade, I recommend Robert Sapolsky's very readable book *Why Zebras Don't Get Ulcers*.[29] Many diseases that are pervasive in today's society are directly attributable to how our bodies respond to our daily stress experiences. Long-term exposure to excessive stress will seriously compromise your immune system. Stress can, in fact, cause us to store unwanted and unnecessary fat. For this reason, we should work hard to reduce our stress experiences. In

---

[29] Robert M. Sapolsky, *Why Zebra Don't Get Ulcers*, 3rd ed. (New York: Henry Holt, 2004).

addition, exercise, a good diet, and adequate rest are essential to help your body recover.

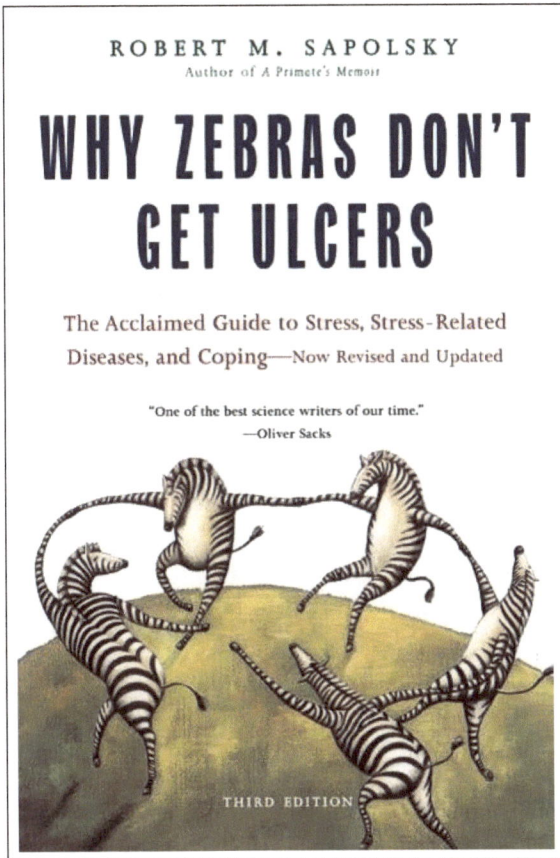

ROBERT M. SAPOLSKY
Author of *A Primate's Memoir*

WHY ZEBRAS DON'T GET ULCERS

The Acclaimed Guide to Stress, Stress-Related Diseases, and Coping—Now Revised and Updated

"One of the best science writers of our time."
—Oliver Sacks

THIRD EDITION

Stress from mental work, physical activities, and our all-to-frequent fight-or-flight incidents are all stacked on top of one another. Your brain/body system can deal with a finite amount of stress. The pollen in the air, the deadline at your job, the work you did helping a friend move, and the hour you spent stuck in rush-hour traffic all combine to bring down the brain/body system. When this happens, you will not be the exceptional athlete you are designed to be. You will not reach your strength and performance potential. Reducing stress in one area will allow you to tolerate additional stress in another area.

The Stress Bucket

All stress is a threat to the brain/body system, and we are, unfortunately, surrounded by stressors. Pollutants in the atmosphere, preservatives in our food, and pressure from our jobs are all stressors. There are many more types of stressors, such as lack of sleep or poor sleep quality, worry about our finances or the security of our future, and eating too much highly refined or poor-quality food.

Another type of stressor, which may not be immediately obvious, can be the poor quality of our movement or the uncertainty of where we are in space. When we don't know where we are or how to accurately move our limbs, we cannot effectively avoid danger or find food. To the brain/body system, this is a very big issue. Poor movement threatens our survival. The brain's primary function is to ensure our survival. Poor movement is therefore a threat to the brain/body system.

The brain/body system must deal with all these various types of stresses. You may have a higher capacity for tolerating stress today than yesterday, or your capacity might be lower. Someone else may have more or less capacity than you do. Each of us has a different ability to handle stress, and it changes from day to day, week to week, and year to year.

We need to have exertion and physical activity in our lives. However, exercise is also a stress. We must also provide the brain with new challenges. This mental work is a different type of stress. Pollutants, lack of sleep, and arguments are yet other types of stress. Some of these threats to our brain/body system are necessary to make us better, and others are bad for us but are simply unavoidable. What can we do with this information about the variety of stresses to which we are being subjected?

One very valuable image for understanding how the brain deals with the stress we experience is a concept called *the stress bucket.*

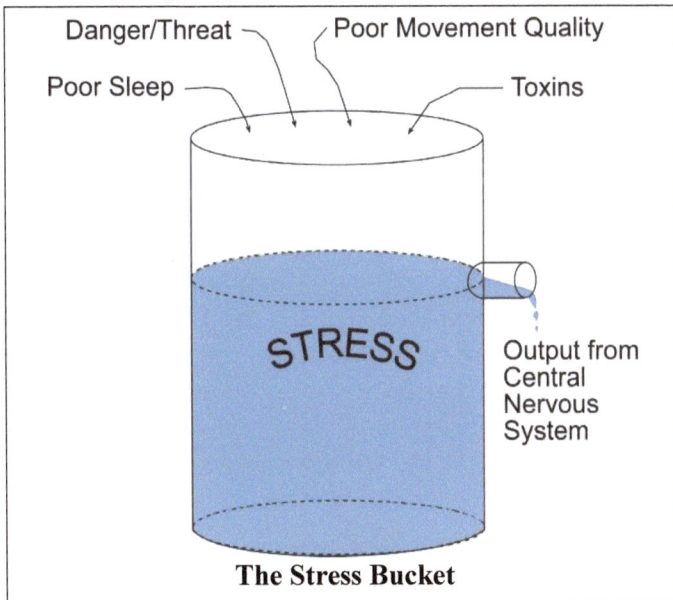

The Stress Bucket

Let's assume you have the capacity to handle five gallons of stress. Imagine that we have a five-gallon bucket with a "Stress" label on the side of it.

Let's start filling up this bucket. First, we pour in one gallon of stress because you are not sleeping well. You stay up too late watching television or working on your computer, and when you finally go to bed, you cannot turn off your inner voice. When you eventually go to sleep, you sleep OK until around two in the morning, when you wake up, use the toilet, and then lie in bed thinking about the workday ahead. Nighttime is when we are supposed to recharge our physical and mental capacities. This is when our memories are formed. When you don't sleep well, you wake up in a fatigued state with reduced abilities to handle stress.

Next, let's pour in one gallon of stress because you live near petrochemical plants that are emitting toxic chemicals by the ton—all day, every day. These toxins enter your lungs and your eyes and require the body to work harder to remove these elements and to clean out your system. Your lungs, kidneys, and liver are working overtime to rid yourself of these materials.

Now, let's pour in two gallons of stress because of your job. Your job can be a significant source of stress. In your case, your boss and clients are demanding, and you feel that you cannot do enough work in the allotted time. You are spending all day in a seated position, staring at a computer monitor. The lack of quality movement, the compromised breathing associated with sitting, and the strain on your eyes all contribute to the stress on your system.

Your stress bucket now has four gallons of stress in it. You have the capacity for one more gallon of stress before you overflow. Now suppose you have a 10K run you are training for, and you are running farther and farther each day. These runs can start to fill up your stress bucket. If, during this period, your child gets sick and you have a fight with your wife, then your stress bucket may overflow. When this happens, the brain will give you some feedback that you have exceeded your stress capacity. How does it do this?

It would be great if the brain would simply tell you that you need more sleep or need to breathe some fresh air, but the brain is a poor communicator. It will incessantly try to tell you something, but figuring out what it is trying to say requires patience and careful listening.

There are many ways the brain can communicate with you. It may make you feel tired or reduce your ability to concentrate at work. You might feel stiff or have limited range of motion in some joints. You may not run as well during your practice sessions. Your balance may be compromised or not as good as usual. You might have less strength than last week. And best of all, you might start feeling achy or notice an increase in an old, recurrent pain. The takeaway from this stress bucket imagery is this: if you are currently under more stress than the brain thinks you should be handling, then you might be weak or experience chronic pain. You can often become stronger or reduce your chronic pain simply by taking some of the stress out of your bucket. Any stress will do. If you get more sleep, then you will probably be stronger. If you save some money so that you aren't constantly worrying about what would happen if you lost your job, then you might have better balance. And if you learn to move better and thereby reduce your fear of falling, then you might reduce or eliminate that nagging pain in your neck that has been bothering you for the past two years.

> *Too much stress can cause your bucket to overflow. The result will be pain or poor performance.*

I explain this to my clients every day. I know it is a difficult concept to integrate into our paradigm. Imagine that you are becoming ill, or you drank too much and went to bed very late. How will you feel? *Everything* will be worse. Your vision, your balance, and your strength and endurance will all be compromised. And you are quite likely to have aches or an increase in chronic pain.

With this analogy, it is important to note that we are not simply trying to reduce the amount of stress in the bucket until we don't have any more. This is impossible and undesirable. We are adaptive creatures. If we have less stress day after day, then eventually our stress bucket will become smaller, and we will be less able to handle the problems that life throws at us. We do want stress or challenges in our lives. But we want just enough that it causes our ability to deal with stressors to increase. We don't want so much stress that it causes the system to begin to shut down. We don't want or need chronic pain or fatigue, poor balance, stiffness, or weakness.

We don't want an infinite amount of sleep. We want just the right amount that will make us perform our best. Too much physical activity can cause the brain/body system too much stress and overload it. For most people, this is unlikely. We want the right amount of exercise to make us better. Too little will not help us improve, and too much might break us. As we apply stress from physical training, over time, we can become stronger and more resilient. In other words, we will become more resistant to the stress of physical performance. Similarly, challenging our mind will improve its function. Ultimately, the size of our stress bucket will increase so that we are better able to handle life's demands.

Some stressors, however, should be eliminated as much as possible because they simply don't help us become better. Pollutants, poor-quality sleep, and a bad diet will not help you become the exceptional athlete you want to be. Taking a little more poison each day in the hope that we will build up a tolerance to it may not be a wise life plan.

Paradigm Shift

Early in the Z-Health training program, the student will learn a set of exercises we call *high-payoff drills*. A couple of these drills involve the feet and ankles. Why? As I mentioned in chapter 1, shoes restrict the movement of our feet and ankles and compromise the quality sensory input from them that the brain wants. We have maps in our brain of our body parts. When the brain maps become fuzzy or unclear, this poses a threat to our survival. Improving the quality of our brain maps reduces the threat or stress on our brains.

The proper function of our feet and ankles is a requirement to ensure our survival. Most people do very little to help their feet and ankles become strong and mobile. As a result, we don't move athletically. This is a threat, and the brain is unhappy about this.

Many people work out or exercise week after week and have little to show for their effort. They do not get better, stronger, or faster. Now I know that improving our brain maps and reducing the threat on the brain will make us better. In almost every case, let's say 90 percent, I have seen my clients improve simply by spending a few minutes working on ankle mobility. What form do these improvements take? They will become more flexible, their balance will improve, and they become stronger. Everything improves.

We have been conditioned by television and magazines to believe that exercise is good for us. And from the media's onslaught, we believe we know what kind of exercise we should be doing. This means we must lift weights, run on a treadmill, attend aerobics classes, and the like. These types of exercises and training are not necessarily bad for you. Although they might be. We must also maintain our ability to move well.

All the joints in our body are supposed to move throughout their normal ranges of motion. When we can no longer move a joint or cannot feel where our body is in space, the brain interprets this sensory-motor amnesia as a threat to our survival. Too much threat will cause us to perform poorly, become weak, or experience pain. The usual result of even a small reduction in threat and stress on the brain/body system is that we will get better. We will become more efficient athletes. And our chronic pain will decrease or disappear.

Now I know that the very best thing I can do for my clients is to improve their movement skills. In my group exercise classes, we might do many things during a training session such as swinging a kettlebell, performing bodyweight exercises, running, and practicing Tae Kwon Do. But now I will always "sneak in" some quality movement skill training because I know that this is what the client really needs most. The client might view this portion of the training session as "rest" because it usually doesn't involve heavy weights, high repetitions, a pounding heart, or panting. This is OK by me. I have found that most clients feel they are not getting a workout and they are not improving if the only thing we do is work on mobility. Clients are happy if they are tired and sweaty. I am happy if they leave our training sessions healthy, more mobile, and more athletic.

Chapter 7: Learning—Everything Is a Skill

We begin life with essentially a blank slate. We can learn whatever language is being spoken in our country and acquire almost any necessary survival abilities required for the region in which we live. Notice that we are not born with these talents, but rather, they are learned through practice and the necessity of our environment. This includes virtually all mental and physical skills.

> *Everything is a skill. All skills can be improved through conscious, repetitive, quality practice.*

Neuroplasticity

Until relatively recently, the scientific community believed that the neural circuitry of the brain developed during adolescence and then became fixed during our twenties. We now know that this is untrue. We are capable of learning new languages, creating new memories, and developing new physical movement skills for our entire lives. The brain is constantly adapting—growing new neural circuits and discarding unused ones. This is the relatively new field of *neuroplasticity*.

This is great news for victims of strokes or physical brain trauma. Using techniques pioneered by Dr. Bach-y-Rita and Dr. Edward Taub called *constraint-induced therapy* (or CI therapy) patients very often can completely regain lost function. However, just like learning to tie knots with your toes, this is very difficult work. But it is possible to regain function if the desire is great enough.

Not only is this neuroplasticity of the brain good news for stroke victims but also good news for you! It means that you can continue to learn new skills, including movement skills, throughout your life. You are never too old to grow new neural connections and to rewire the brain. In fact, the brain is constantly changing whether or not you want it to.

Your brain is constantly receiving information from the sensory inputs throughout your body and is processing this information. The brain uses this data to create concepts of where we are, how we move, and what we are capable of doing. Because this process is happening all day, every day, we are unaware of the small changes. But these small changes add up over time.

Suppose you have an injury to your ankle. The pain you experience and the time of nonuse during the healing process will cause you to make some compensatory changes in your movement patterns. When your ankle is fully healed and pain free, you go on about your business and assume everything is wonderful. But is it? You may have slightly changed the position of your ankle during gait. This will have an effect on the forces that travel throughout your body. Remember that the most important exercise you are likely doing is walking. There are huge adaptive forces at work every day as you simply walk about. The change to your ankle as a result of your inadequately rehabilitated ankle injury can have far-reaching effects. Everything is connected: your ankles, your knees, your hips, your spine, your shoulders, and more.

Inputs from your entire body are integrated into the brain and interpreted to create an image of who we are and how we move. When we have a body part, in this case, an ankle, that is not moving as we think it is moving, there is a mismatch between reality and our perception. For us to perform as exceptional athletes, we must know the truth about where we are and what we are capable of. The lack of ability to move a body part accurately or to clearly understand its position in space, or sensory motor amnesia, reduces our athleticism.

Every one of our movements causes many areas of the brain to fire. Each movement is a complex collection of motor neural outputs, visualization or recollection of previous events, and the processing of ongoing sensory inputs. When one or more parts of the system are not accurately represented and we use the system in this way over and over again, we make new unathletic neural circuits, and eventually, these movement patterns become more permanent.

This is why the magic of Z-Health makes possible the often-immediate elimination of chronic pain. As soon as we clarify the movement map or the sensory input from an area that has sensory motor amnesia, the brain perceives that we have become more athletic. We understand more accurately where we are and how we can move. Improved movement reduces the threat to our survival. As a result, the brain rewards us with increased range of motion, more strength, better balance, and reduced pain.

> *Thanks to its neuroplastic properties, we can change the structure of our brain.*

Brain Stories

In chapter 3, you were introduced to Norman Doidge and his book, *The Brain That Changes Itself*. One of the stories he relates is about Pedro Bach-y-Rita. He was a poet and a scholar who, in 1959 at age sixty-five, had a severe stroke. Half his face and half his body were paralyzed. He was unable to speak. The medical profession did all the usual things for stroke victims, including trying to teach him how to use the limited function that had not been lost due to the stroke. Eventually, they pronounced that he would not be able to speak, walk, or feed himself. His son George took his dad to Mexico and began by teaching his father to crawl. In other words, he started at the beginning and retrained his father.

Pedro worked diligently at his rehabilitation and regained the ability to walk, type, and speak. He returned to full-time work at City College in New York. He worked there until he retired at age seventy. At age seventy-two, Pedro died from a heart attack while climbing in the mountains in Bogota, Columbia.

Pedro's other son, Dr. Paul Bach-y-Rita (1934–2006), being a good scientist, requested an autopsy be performed on his father, so he could learn something about the stroke and his miraculous, subsequent recovery. What he discovered was astonishing.

A large portion of the brain had been destroyed by the stroke, including most of the brain stem. This is the area of the brain responsible for our basic movement skills. Yet, amazingly, through very difficult work, Pedro had been able to rewire his own brain and to regain much of its lost function![30]

---

[30] Doidge, *The Brain That Changes Itself*, 22–3.

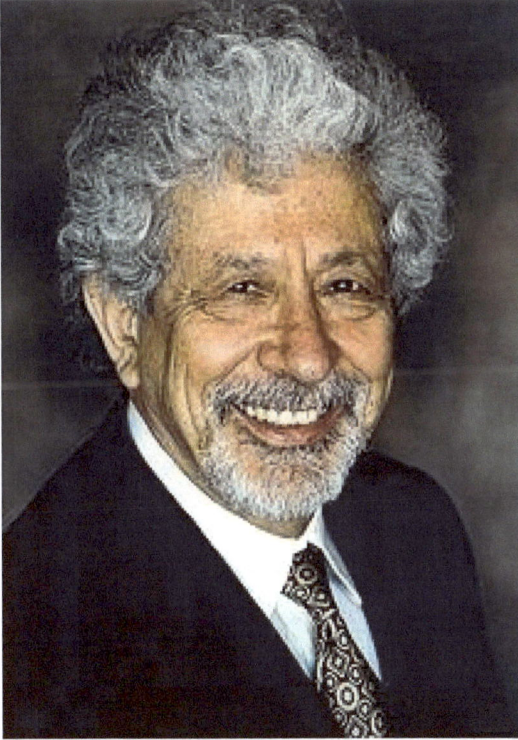

Dr. Paul Bach-y-Rita

Another story about the amazing power of the brain's ability to restructure itself is about a device called the *BrainPort*. Once again we hear about the amazing Dr. Paul Bach-y-Rita. His knowledge of the brain's neuroplastic properties led him to theorize that any area of the brain could be used to process any sensory input. In other words, one type of sensory input could be substituted for another. The brain would then determine how to process this substitute input information.

To test this theory, he connected a camera to a grid of vibrating plates mounted to the back of a chair. The camera's image was converted into electrical signals that could be felt as vibrations on the back of someone sitting in the chair. When he brought in a blind person and connected everything up, something amazing happened. The camera and plates allowed the blind person to "see." The image was very crude due to the resolution or number of pixels, but the person could identify objects and even detect motion.

This initial work was done in the 1960s. In the 1990s, Dr. Bach-y-Rita began looking at the tongue as a better site for connecting the camera's output to the brain's input system. The BrainPort device is a direct result of these initial experiments. It turns out that the tongue has a large quantity of sensitive neurons able to detect small signals. By using the tongue as the sensory input, a higher resolution was possible. A smaller camera was also employed that could fit on the user's forehead. The output device was also shrunken to become a small, postage stamp-sized rectangle. The image resolution was now increased to four hundred pixels or more.

The new output device was then placed on the user's tongue, causing a sensation somewhat like a bubbling or fizzy feeling. Using this newest version of the BrainPort has allowed a blind person to pick up objects, play tic-tac-toe, climb rock walls, and many more activities that sighted people take for granted. As an extreme example, Erik Weihenmayer became the first blind person to climb Mount Everest using the BrainPort device. This is just too amazing to be true—but it is. Blind people can now see by putting a camera on their heads and a sensor in their mouths. Our brain's adaptive abilities are extraordinary. The FDA approved the BrainPort V100 device for sale in America in June 2015, and it is currently available by prescription only.

The Learning Zone
Learning a new skill, whether it is a physical movement skill or a skill involving memory and logic or imagination, creates new neural connections. We are essentially

rewiring our brain through the acquisition of new skills. We get better at those things we constantly do, including skill acquisition. The brain will remain more plastic or pliable if we challenge it daily. Recall that the brain hates boredom and loves novelty, activation, and fuel. As with most things, having a goal or a target will help us achieve the optimal amount of stimulation so that we get a little better every day. Here, our goal will be *the learning zone.*

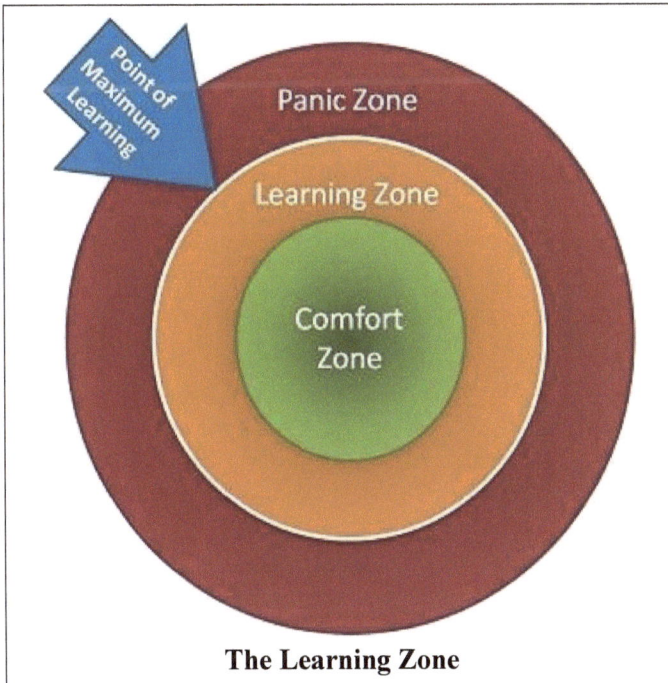

The Learning Zone

Let's look first at *the comfort zone.* Imagine that you have a favorite lounge chair in a warm, dimly lit room. Your chair is very comfortable. You have a nice, foamy cup of hot chocolate or your other favorite beverage to sip on. You are wearing your cherished pajamas and your fuzzy slippers. Your favorite music is playing. You are in heaven. If you spend too much time in your comfort zone, then you will soon find that it is no longer really comfortable. You will want something different to drink. Lounging in your chair will become annoying. You will develop an irresistible urge to get up and move around in the sunshine. Your comfort zone will shrink when you spend time there.

When we experience sufficient novelty and challenge, we leave the comfort zone and enter the learning zone. Here, we have stimulation, we are growing new neural connections, and we are improving. This is the place where we, like children, like to play. It is interesting, challenging, and far from boring. It doesn't seem like work, and we don't want it to end. Children love to play tag. One kid runs away, and another one tries to catch him or her. The end result is usually two or more sweaty kids. But they don't see this as exercise or work. This phenomenon is not limited to children. This is why we have invented so many games: basketball, football, tennis, soccer. This entertainment or stimulation is not limited to physical activities. We can also amuse ourselves with mental activities such as chess, board or card games, Rubik's cubes, and the like. Various types of sensory stimulation can also put us into the learning zone. We like massages, swinging, riding a bicycle, jumping on a trampoline, or even skydiving.

This leads us to consider the third zone, *the panic (or danger) zone*. While skydiving might be thrilling, exciting, or invigoration to one person, another individual might become ill and experience an intense anxiety attack. Too much stimulation, novelty, or challenge might not make us better and may cause us to shut down. When things become excessive, our fight-or-flight response takes over and can, over time, actually cause physical damage to the brain/body system. Recall our discussion of the stress bucket. Too much of a good thing is often just too much.

We have now divided our world into three zones: the comfort zone, the learning zone, and the panic zone. Too much time in the comfort zone will make us worse. The same is true of the panic zone. We will get better when we spend most of our time in the learning zone. Everyone's learning zone is unique. What will make you better might be too intense for someone else. Similarly, what might be interesting and challenging for someone else might be well within your comfort zone, and it will not adequately stimulate you.

Our goal in describing these three zones is to help identify how you can improve your physical or mental skills. In other words, how do we make the brain happy? How do we get better? Recall that when the brain/body system gets better, *everything* gets better. We can improve our ability to acquire or sharpen skills by better identifying our goal. Our goal is to spend more time in the learning zone. But we can do even better than this. Our goal is to spend time in the learning zone but as close to the panic zone as possible. This means we want as much challenge and stimulus as possible without going over the top.

How do we know if we go too far? Simple. We get worse. Our strength goes down. Our range of motion decreases. This is how we know where the panic zone begins. Back off just a little from this level of challenge and return to your activity once again. Eventually, you will find that sweet spot in the learning zone where you will make the greatest and fastest improvements in your skill acquisition. The three things you can readily adjust in your training to help you find this sweet spot are (1) range of motion, (2) load or intensity, and (3) speed. A greater range of motion or a higher load can increase the challenge. Reducing these factors enough will usually move you back into the learning zone. Speed is a bit different. Sometimes doing things more slowly may be easier, or it may be more difficult depending on the activity. As an example, try the one-minute push-up. Take thirty seconds to descend and thirty seconds to come back up. This will probably be quite challenging for you.

Just as spending time in your comfort zone will cause it to shrink in size, training or playing in your learning zone near the edge of the panic zone will also cause the boundaries to change. Your abilities will increase, your brain/body system will get better, and the learning zone will expand. You will be able to challenge yourself more and more while still remaining in the learning zone. What once was far too difficult for you to do is now well within your capabilities.

The LTAD Model

Every country wants its athletes to bring home lots of medals from the Olympic games. To this end, Canada started looking at the history of successful athletes, and from that work, they came up with the Long-Term Athletic Development (LTAD) model. The Canadian Sport for Life Society was formed in 2005. This group determined that top-level athletes shared some common histories of development. For example, most (but not all) top athletes were exposed to a wide variety of sports and a range of playful activities during their early childhoods. These years allowed the athletes to form a broad base of quality movement skills that could later be integrated to form a solid foundation for their chosen sports. It takes many years and thousands of hours of dedicated practice to become a world-class athlete. Being genetically gifted will help, but it is not enough. You will probably also be unsuccessful if you are practicing the wrong things or practicing them at the wrong time.

The LTAD model divides athletes and their skills into two groups.

- Early specialization (figure skating, diving, gymnastics, etc.)

- Late specialization (tennis, field sports, skiing, basketball, cycling, etc.)

For some sports, if you don't start training early enough, then you will simply run out of time. This is an early specialization sport. For example, Olympic gymnast Nadia Comaneci was fourteen years old when she scored a perfect 10 for her routine. To reach this level, she simply *had* to begin training hard and specifically on gymnastics at a very young age.

To achieve excellence in other sports, such as those in the late specialization group, the athlete may need to acquire a broad base of skills and to learn to rapidly process the sensory input from hands, feet, vision, and more, prior to focusing on their chosen sports.

The LTAD model is not only concerned with the development of Olympic athletes but also with ensuring that people remain mobile, healthy, and athletic into later stages of life. All of us are athletes, even if we never make it to the Olympics. Even Olympic athletes should have a high quality of life after their moments of glory. Whether the sport we are trying to master is an early or late specialization activity, there are stages through which the athlete should progress. The following are the seven basic stages of the LTAD model:

- Stage 1: Active Start (0–6 years)
- Stage 2: FUNdamentals (girls 6–8, boys 6–9)
- Stage 3: Learn to Train (girls 8–11, boys 9–12)
- Stage 4: Train to Train (girls 11–15, boys 12–16)
- Stage 5: Train to Compete (girls 15–21, boys 16–23)
- Stage 6: Train to Win (girls 18+, boys 19+)

- Stage 7: Active for Life (any age participant)[31]

Stages 1, 2, and 3 are about the development of basic physical skills and learning to enjoy being active as a part of daily life. The focus is on overall movement skill development and the integration of mental and emotional abilities.

Stages 4, 5, and 6 are about the development of elite athletic skills and are centered on physical and mental training and learning how to compete. Focus on a specific sport occurs here. Additional loading, such as free weights, might begin to appear as part of the training in these stages. Training intensity increases in order to support progress and to prepare for intensely competitive situations.

Based on this model, there is an optimal time for exposure to certain types of training. For most sports activities, it is essential that involvement begin with fun, enjoyment, and excitement. There should be a certain thrill associated with the activity. In other words, for kids, it must be something they want to do.

Once they are really interested in the sport or activity, we can teach them how to become better at the necessary skills. Because they enjoy the sport, they will be willing to invest time in learning technique and deep practice. Their work will not be simply drudgery but something they will enthusiastically do in order to more fully enjoy their activities. Most of their involvement during this phase will still be play, but they will want to perform better in order to have more fun.

As the athlete matures, he or she will be ready to engage in competition. This phase requires that the athlete learn to

---

[31] "LTAD Stages," Canadian Sport for Life Society, Accessed February 24, 2017, http://canadiansportforlife.ca/learn-about-canadian-sport-life/ltad-stages.

control some of the mental aspects of the sport and to learn to evaluate and react to the competition's performance. Competition at this level is still fun. Winning is not everything but another activity to help the athlete mature. Enjoyment and social interactions are a part of this developmental process.

With a strong basis in love for the activity, sports-specific skills, and knowledge of competitive nuances, the athlete is now ready to learn to win. This phase requires more intensive training and a willingness to push hard for improvement.

Hopefully, these athletes will acquire a desire for quality movement skills and a healthy lifestyle that will serve them well once the competitive years are behind them. We can stay athletic throughout our lives. This will help us remain happy and healthy and allow us to engage in a wide variety of enjoyable activities with our families and friends for many years.

The main reason I have included this description of the LTAD model is that it also encourages a paradigm shift. Many people in America live vicariously through their children. Suppose Dad wanted to be a baseball player, or he simply loves the sport. He might even have a son who really seems to be both interested in and good at baseball. So, Dad, wanting to give his boy the very best chance of succeeding (and getting the ever-elusive multimillion-dollar pro contract), starts teaching him baseball at the age of three. Then the boy is put in T-ball, and Dad is practicing with him on weekends. You get the picture.

According to the LTAD model, specializing in a sport at a very young age can deprive the child of the requisite exposure to many other necessary skills. While these other skills, such as dribbling, climbing, jumping, or wrestling, may not seem relevant to the sport of baseball, they in fact develop a much-needed broad base of physical movement skills. Without this foundation, the athlete is unlikely to reach his or her full potential.

Another paradigm shift that can come from the study of the LTAD model is that of competition. Putting very young athletes into competitive situations at too early an age deprives them of quality training on the basics. Kids must learn to love physical activity and their sports. Then they must learn how to train and to develop the discipline to do this work. Recall the discussion of deep, deliberate practice from chapter 3. It takes around ten thousand hours of practice to achieve mastery or to reach an expert level. If athletes focus too much on competition prior to significant quality training and practice time, then they will learn to compete with poor skills. These athletes will learn to compete by working around their compensations and inadequacies instead of addressing and correcting them. Athletes will be much more likely to be highly competitive if they learn how to train and to apply several years to this part of their development.

Paradigm Shift

For decades, I have taught group Tae Kwon Do classes. These classes usually had between ten and thirty students. About a decade ago, I began teaching group kettlebell classes. In the beginning, these classes usually also had between ten and thirty students. In every class, there were gifted students, average students, and below-average students. I felt I needed to provide challenge for the talented athletes, or they would leave. Further, I was sure that pushing the average clients to excel was a good thing. This would help them get in shape and increase their strength and stamina. As for the below-average students, I would do my best to scale the exercises or training to something that they could safely do. However, no one wants to be the person at the back of the class doing a scaled-down exercise. So, those students with poor movement, skill deficits, and generally unathletic movement qualities would either push themselves harder than everyone else in a vain attempt to keep up, or they would all too quickly abandon the program.

What I now know is that we are each exactly where we are. What will make each of us better is unique to us, and it depends on where we are right now. If I can do ten push-ups, then doing one push-up is not very challenging and doing fifty push-ups might be too much. Some people cannot do one push-up. Some people can do fifty push-ups. And this analysis is only about push-ups. Every movement skill for each individual must be evaluated in terms of strength, endurance, speed, and range of motion. The training challenge presented, if it is to encourage improvement in the athlete, must be at just the right level near the edge of the learning zone.

Group classes are exciting. There is an energy that comes from a group of like-minded individuals pushing themselves toward a common goal. We will each work harder and attempt things we might not try on our own. We receive satisfaction from our own achievements and from watching those around us break through barriers and achieve new performance levels.

However, what I now know to be the case is that group classes can be a recipe for failure on a couple of levels. First, many people will not receive enough challenge, and therefore, they will not make the progress that will prove rewarding to them. These people will likely move on and hopefully find a more exciting and fun activity. Second, *most* people will find one or more of the drills or movements performed during the group class to be too difficult. They will attempt them anyway. Either they will continue to practice the movement with compensations and poor quality, thereby further ingraining these inefficient movements, or the load will be too great, and they will run a significant risk of injury.

The paradigm shift I had to make is this: in order to improve, you must challenge yourself physically and mentally in a variety of ways, but the level of these challenges should be whatever is required to make you better. Not more. Not less. Therefore, most people will improve faster when training alone or with a coach or with a small number of equally skilled athletes. I have not always been doing my students and clients the best service I could by running large-group classes.

Chapter 8: Change

Change is difficult. We are much more comfortable when things remain the same, and we think (almost always erroneously) that we know what tomorrow will bring. To continue with the status quo is much easier and uses much less energy. We don't need to think too hard or unnecessarily exert ourselves. Our brains, being concerned primarily with survival, prefer to conserve energy. But if we want to grow, then we simply *must* change.

How do we make a change in ourselves? First, we must determine if there is something we would like to change. Until this happens, we will continue doing the same thing we did yesterday. We will continue doing that same old exercise that we have become quite good at but which doesn't make us better. Once again, tomorrow, we will hope that magically we will begin to improve. It is unwise to do the same thing over and over and hope that the outcome will suddenly be different.

In this stage of our fledgling transformational process, we haven't even thought about making a change. We haven't identified *the thing* that would be a candidate for change. There is usually (but not always) a significant event that causes a spark and shines a little bit of light on the thing we want to change. When this happens, we see the world slightly differently — we see that we would like something to be different.

When that happens, we must *believe* in the possibility that this change could occur. In other words, we must have hope. This is a key element in Paradigm Z: we must believe (and therefore have the expectation) that we can successfully change ourselves. Why is this both necessary and possible? Because you and I are constantly changing anyway. To improve simply requires that we arrange things so that this daily, ongoing change is a positive one that carries us a little bit closer to our goal every day. In this way, we can get a little better each day.

Stages of Change

In order to successfully make a change, each person must go through stages. As a coach, I must help the client (or persuade him or her) to move through these stages. The effort to make the change is made by the client, and I am the facilitator. The following is an example of what these stages of change might look like:

- Change from resisting to listening.

- Go from listening to considering.

- Shift from considering to willing to do.

- Change from willing to do to actually doing.

- Move from doing to glad they did and to continue doing.[32]

We are where we are—physically, mentally, and emotionally. We cannot jump from the ability to struggle through a single push-up on our knees to the new talent of performing a one-arm pushup. Any significant change we make requires us to go through a paradigm shift, and we must sequentially go through stages similar to those outlined earlier. One of the best ways to help our clients make the difficult leap from one stage to another is to listen to what they say and to ask them questions. Ultimately, progress will be made when the *client* says he or she is ready to make a change—not before. Mark Goulston's book *Just Listen* is an excellent introduction to yet another skill set I needed to acquire.[33] This listening

---

[32] Mark Goulston, *Just Listen: Discover the Secret to Getting Through to Absolutely Anyone* (New York: AMACOM, 2010), 8.
[33] Ibid.

skill now allows me to better help people move toward their desired future.

When we carefully listen to our clients, they will recognize the attention we are giving them and usually will be appreciative. Having developed the necessary rapport, we will be able to ask the appropriate and sometimes difficult questions without coming across as threatening or demeaning. Exceptional listening skills will also enable us to glean clues about the client's motivation for change and what some of his or her barriers to progress may be. If we truly want to help others improve, then successful listening is the first step.

The second step is identifying where they are and what stage they are currently in. We rarely get to skip steps in our development. We must sit, then crawl, then walk, and then run. This logic applies to our stages of change, both for us personally and for those whom we are trying to help make positive changes.

James Prochaska, John Norcross, and Carlo DiClemente's book, *Changing for Good,* describes the transtheoretical model of change. This model was developed from research that indicated all people who are successful in making significant changes go through six specific stages.

- Precontemplation
- Contemplation
- Preparation
- Action
- Maintenance
- Termination[34]

---

[34] James O. Prochaska, John C. Norcross, and Carlo C. DiClemente, *Changing for Good: A Revolutionary Six-Stage Program for*

Steps in this sequence cannot be skipped if the long-term change is to be successful. Therefore, an understanding of these stages can help us avoid that mistake.

I have introduced you to two models that show we must move through specific stages in our process of change. Another somewhat different model I encountered years ago comes from Bruce Lee. He describes these stages or actions to be taken as Buddhism's Eightfold Path.

1. *Right views:* You must clearly see what is wrong.

2. *Right purpose:* You must decide to be cured.

3. *Right speech:* You must speak so as to aim at being cured.

4. *Right conduct:* You must act.

5. *Right vocation:* Your livelihood must not conflict with your therapy.

6. *Right effort:* The therapy must go forward at the "staying speed," the critical velocity that can be sustained.

7. *Right awareness:* You must feel it and think about it incessantly.

8. *Right concentration:* Learn how to contemplate with the deep mind.[35]

Regardless of the stages of change model you choose to embrace, both you and your client are somewhere along the path from desiring a change to moving toward this new future to fully realizing a new and better person.

Motivational Interviewing

Overcoming Bad Habits and Moving Your Life Positively Forward (New York: William Morrow, 1994), 39.

[35] Bruce Lee, *Tao of Jeet Kune Do* (Santa Clarita, CA: Ohara, 1975), 9.

One of the most difficult moments in my Z-Health journey was when I learned that it was not all about me. Who would want to discover this? For decades, I had been teaching Tae Kwon Do. My job (or so I thought) was to *tell* the students what to do. After all, I was the expert. If they didn't listen, then it was their own fault that they didn't improve. What I learned was that, most often, if you want to help someone make a change, then telling him or her what to do is not the best approach. We do not believe what others tell us, and we will almost always argue against what we are told. Who do we believe? Who is the *only* person we really believe? Ourselves. As a result, I learned that if I truly wanted to be a better teacher and coach, then I had to face the fact that I could be a much better listener. I needed to change the way I communicated with my clients. In fact, I also needed to change the way I talked to myself.

One of the first steps in helping others make a change is building a rapport with them. In order to do this, I needed to learn to listen better. The client must *know* that you are interested in him or her and that you truly want to help. It is much more important to be interested than to be interesting. As I began to learn, it *could not* be about me if I wanted to help them. What *I* know is not the most important thing. What *I* can do isn't the most important thing. The thing that determines the client's ability to improve is where the client is, what the client is thinking, and the next small sustainable change that the client can make toward a better future.

The next step is to identify where the client is. What stage of change is he or she in? To do this, I needed to know the stages of change and to be able to identify them—because my goal and my job is to help the client successfully progress from one stage to the next. Sounds simple, doesn't it?

It really isn't.

The key to progressing from this point forward is to realize that people only believe what *they* say. Although I may have lots of training, knowledge, and experience, it really doesn't matter what I *tell* the client to do or why he or she should do it. What matters is that the client decides and tells himself or herself or tells me that he or she wants to change, what he or she wants to change, how he or she will change, and why he or she wants to do this. Then the client will believe it. We trust ourselves, and we believe what we say. And we don't like to lie to ourselves. As soon as we hear ourselves say it out loud, in our minds, we think, "Yep, that's true!" We need to find a way to get our client to say the right thing. I can hear the old me lecturing the client and saying, "You shouldn't eat two pieces of cheesecake every day." And I can see the client nodding his head in agreement. But, inside his head, he was probably saying, "This guy doesn't know what I should do." We must get the client to argue for the change he or she wants.

One way to do this is to say things that are untrue. A good deal of rapport is required for this method of communication. For example, what will happen if I say, "If you work out a lot and the pieces are small, then you could probably eat two or even three pieces of cheesecake each day"? The likely response would be "I wouldn't need to work out so much if I ate less cheesecake" or "If I eat three pieces of cheesecake every day, then there is no way I could work out enough." Now the client is arguing *for* the desired change.

When I was in my early teens, I asked my father to teach me how to play guitar. He told me that I couldn't learn to play guitar because it was difficult and required patience and dedication. I said to myself, "I will show him. I *can* and I *will* learn to play guitar!" Within a few months, he asked me to show him how I was able to do some things on the guitar that he was unable to do. Desire and commitment are essential in order to make changes. Sometimes, the best way to help your clients is to agree that they cannot succeed. Then they will argue that they *can* succeed.

Another tool for getting the client to argue for the desired change is the *change ruler*. This technique works like this. Imagine that the client has a desire to add more fresh vegetables to his or her diet. In your conversation with your client, you could say, "You know that you need to eat more vegetables." However, this will cause your client's internal dialogue to argue against eating more vegetables. Instead, we want the client to argue *for* the desired change.

Here's how the change ruler would be applied. Ask the client, on a scale of one to ten, how he or she would rate his or her desire to eat more vegetables, with one being uninterested and ten being extremely desirable. Let's assume the client says three. The follow-up question would be: "Why did you choose three instead of two?" Immediately, the client is put into a position where he or she must think about why he or she *wants* to eat vegetables, and the client must verbalize this. Even if you know this trick is being performed on you, profound changes will occur, and you will start to talk yourself into changing.

Instant Influence by Michael Pantalon is an excellent and readable introduction to the skill of motivational interviewing.[36] Doctors working in emergency rooms often see the same patient repeatedly for excessive drinking or drug abuse. Wouldn't it be better if instead of treating only the patient's symptoms the doctor could help the patient

---

[36] Michael V. Pantalon, *Instant Influence: How to Get Anyone to Do Anything—Fast* (New York: Little Brown, 2011).

change his or her behavior? Here is what Dr. Pantalon says about this process:

> *The ER docs were so successful using my approach that they were able to achieve a nearly 50 percent reduction in drinking among their "alcohol-involved" patients — just from seven-minute conversations. As a result, Instant Influence is now a standard part of care in emergency rooms and in major trauma units across the United States, and medical residents nationwide are required to learn it.*[37]

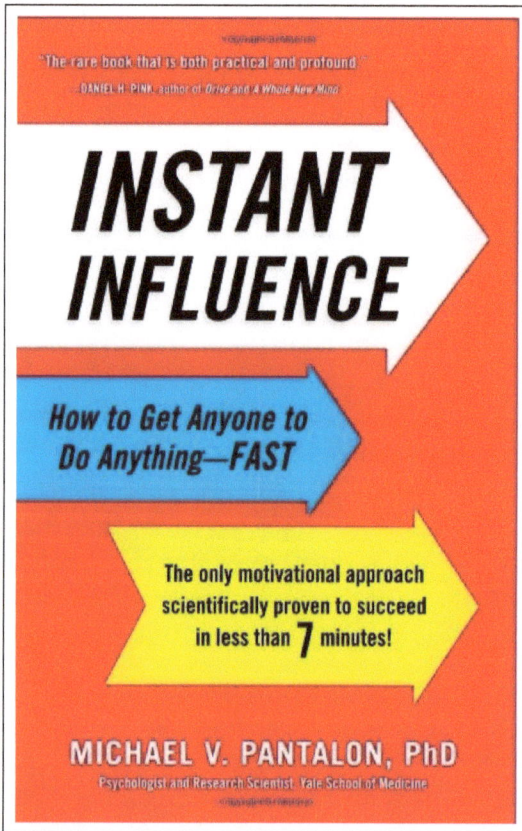

INSTANT INFLUENCE

How to Get Anyone to Do Anything—FAST

The only motivational approach scientifically proven to succeed in less than 7 minutes!

MICHAEL V. PANTALON, PhD
Psychologist and Research Scientist, Yale School of Medicine

---

[37] Ibid., 6.

The following are the six steps or conversational questions that Dr. Pantalon says will help you achieve instant influence:

- Step 1: Why might you change? (Or to influence yourself, why might I change?)

- Step 2: How ready are you to change on a scale from one to ten, where one means "not ready at all" and ten means "totally ready"?

- Step 3: Why didn't you pick a lower number? (Or, if the influencee picked one, either ask the second question again, this time about a smaller step toward change, or ask what would it take for that one to turn into a two.)

- Step 4: Imagine you've changed. What would the positive outcomes be?

- Step 5: Why are those outcomes important to you?

- Step 6: What's the next step, if any?[38]

Using the change ruler strategy in conversation is a skill that must be honed through practice. Your conversation should feel comfortable and natural to both you and the client. One of the great things about the Z-Health courses is that they provide a forum and a safe, supportive environment where you get to practice this method of conversing with various pretend clients. You will be surprised at the effectiveness of this technique, even when others do it to you, and you know they are doing it!

Paradigm Shift

During most of my school years, I acted as a teaching assistant in various courses to help others improve their grades. I always felt that my job was to identify what the

---

[38] Ibid., 5–6.

students didn't know or understand and then to share that information with them. They didn't know what to do, and I would tell them.

I employed the same tactics while teaching Tae Kwon Do. I had the knowledge, and my job was to impart this information to the student. The more knowledge I had, the better instructor I would be, right? Well, not quite.

Now I know that my job as an instructor or coach is not to simply impart my knowledge to the recipient but rather to help him or her change. As an example, suppose the client wants to learn to perform a physical feat such as a one-arm push-up. I regress the exercise to one that the client can perform—perhaps it is a push-up performed on the knees. I impart some wisdom about alignment and form and then I *tell* the client to go home and practice this exercise every other day and instruct him or her to do fifteen repetitions. Does this strategy work? Very rarely.

Instead, the client returns for the next session and says that he or she didn't have time or forgot or some other such excuse. Change, if it is to occur, is up to the client. The client must do the work. In other words, the client *must decide* that he or she wants to make a change, and the client *will* do the work because *he or she* wants to, not because I told the client to do it. The client might do it if I am standing over him or her, pushing him or her to do it. But real, lasting changes occur within each of us, and they happen when it is important to us.

Yes, it is important for the instructor to possess knowledge, experience, and skill. However, communication skills are equally important and perhaps even more essential to success. My job is to determine what the client needs, what the client wants, and where the client currently is. From this information, if I am successfully able to influence the client, then positive changes can occur—but only if the client does the work.

Chapter 9: Exercise

Do you want to move better and become more athletic? Are you working out on a regular basis? Is your training program making you better? If not, then you might consider changing the focus of your practice sessions. Your workouts are not supposed to break you. Rather, they should make you better. Training hard can be good for you, but you should also be smart with your time and effort.

Day after day, week after week, you must be doing something that makes you better. This means that your efforts must be sustainable. If you do not receive some joy or other reward from your training, then it is unlikely to be sustainable.

Fun

Children and animals have something in common. They love to play. Play is fun. Play involves movement and creativity. It engages the body and mind. It is through play that we learn how to move. My young boys always want to run and climb, and they don't think this is unpleasant or tortuous training. On the contrary, play is the *original* exercise. This is how children learn where their bodies are in space and how to move them in a coordinated way. Through play, they also learn what their limitations are. Play is essential *because* it is fun. These pleasant experiences have a powerful influence on the development of our new quality movements. We have returned many times to how emotions are involved in the formation of new neural circuitry. I mentioned Stuart Brown's book, *Play*, in chapter 3. This book offers a more complete discussion of this subject.

What happened to fun and play?

As we enter adulthood, we usually decide that we must work because we need the money. And we must work out because we want to stay in shape. Notice the use of *must* and *work* in both of those sentences. Somewhere between childhood and adulthood, our play turned into exercise, and our fun turned into work. This is problematic. It causes two things to happen. First, most people simply don't want to exercise because it isn't fun. Second, we aren't mentally engaged in the activity. We just want to reach the end of the session, so we can say we did it.

If our physical activity isn't fun, then we will look for any excuse to avoid it. Contrast this with playing a game of volleyball, tennis, or baseball (assuming you would enjoy such an activity). Would you think to yourself, "Do I really have to play?" Or if you were playing in the pool with your friends, would you whine, "When will we be finished?" No. In fact, when we are having fun, time goes by rather quickly. We want the moment to last, and we look forward to the next time we will have the opportunity to experience this feeling of elation and freedom from all worries.

When we view our physical practice as work, very often, we will mentally check out. This is why you see so many people watching TV or reading a book while they are running on a treadmill. They just want to get this torture over with. Or they might be listening to music or an audiobook while running around and around the block.

If our exercise is fun, then we will want to do it. By contrast, we tend to avoid things that are not fun. The brain likes novelty and fun at any age, and it wants to avoid boredom. Do you recall being a child and that the worst fear you had was that you might become bored? New things are exciting. If we truly want to practice quality movement skills and our practice is fun, then we will be mentally engaged in the task. Positive emotion coupled with intense focus helps to quickly create new motor movement patterns in the brain. This is what will make us both feel better and move better.

And isn't one of the things we want to get out of our physical activity the ability to move better? I certainly hope so. Getting better at a physical movement requires that we have a concept or an image of what the desired movement will be. It requires that we execute that movement. And then it requires that we observe the outcome. Did I execute the move as I had envisioned it? Was the timing of all the muscular contractions exactly right? How was my balance? When we are mentally engaged in our physical activity, we will notice how our bodies move, and our inner voice will calm down. When our mind is somewhere else during our exercise, we will continue to practice our poor or compromised movement patterns, and we won't even notice or care. As a result, the quality of our movement will not get better, and we won't be more calm.

Function

The body you have is mostly a direct result of the movements that you have done throughout the course of your life. This is sort of like the statement that form follows function, but it is much more than that.

Your amazing body is extremely adaptable. You can eat meat, live on fish and whale blubber, or be a vegetarian. Humans live in Alaska and northern Siberia as well as in the deserts of the Middle East and in equatorial rain forests. Throughout your life, you are constantly replacing hair, skin, blood cells, muscle tissue, and even bone. You are changing and adapting constantly — all day, every day! This is happening whether you like it or not. You are either gaining muscle or losing muscle. You are growing and reinforcing new neural connections, or they are losing their function.

We can use the body's ability to adapt to change how we function. Suppose you want to be stronger. Regularly challenging yourself to generate significant force can make you stronger. You can do the same thing with endurance and flexibility—choose a sustainable activity that will help you repeatedly push the limits of your endurance and flexibility. Assuming you don't overdo it, you will likely increase both your range of motion and your stamina.

I have spent time with some very strong people. I have a great life. Recall the example in chapter 6 about tearing cards. My skin, bones, muscles, and ligaments must adapt to handle the forces required for this stunt. The real secret is specific hard work and perseverance. But, given time, my body will adapt to provide the desired function, in this case, the ability to tear a deck of cards.

Appearance

Many people are interested in exercise programs solely because they want to "look" a certain way. They want to be attractive to others and to themselves. There is nothing wrong with this. Your reasons for doing whatever you do with your life, including exercise activities, is your business. Hopefully, you will set realistic but challenging goals for yourself. But we must be honest with ourselves. If you are five feet tall, then it is unlikely that you can work hard and become six feet tall.

Take a look at the world around you and the people in it. You will see very skinny and often unhealthy-looking marathon runners. You may see very large and slow-moving weight lifters. You will also see sedentary office workers who are overweight and who move poorly. And you probably know some people who do very little exercise or eat healthy food but still look like lean models.

Much of the way we look is determined at birth. Yet another contributor to our body composition is determined by our food intake. Genetics and nutrition affect the way we look. But you can still look at exceptional athletes and learn something from the types of bodies they possess. Gymnasts look like gymnasts, swimmers look like swimmers, ballet dancers look like ballet dancers, and sprinters look like sprinters.

This knowledge gives us a clue as to how we can achieve the bodies and appearance we want. Choose that group of athletes who look like you want to look and then do what those athletes do. This may not be easy. In fact, it will surely not be easy. All exceptional athletes have changed their bodies through commitment and diligent hard work. But they love their sports. In fact, they view practice and training for their sports as play — as fun. Another great example is tennis players. They are generally lean, they are quick, they move well, and they have good endurance. But they are spending much of their time playing.

This entire discussion may seem obvious. But we see people going to the gym, spending many boring hours on a treadmill, and expecting to develop the body they want. However, if they just look at the treadmills to the left and right, then they will see many unhappy, overweight people with poor movement skills. In spite of the lack of success of their exercise programs, people continue to devote time to this activity. Is your goal to be a stair-climber athlete or a treadmill athlete?

Health
Health and well-being are an often-overlooked objective of our exercise program. (That seems impossible to me as I write it, but I know it to be so.) Many people are so focused on their appearance or their desire to lose weight that they are really not too concerned with becoming healthier. Others are obsessed with improving a specific athletic skill and will push themselves into an unhealthy state while trying to achieve those goals. Of course, some

people are working out just for the cardiovascular benefit. They may be doing this because they want to live longer or (more likely) because the doctor told them they need to do it, and they feel guilty if they don't do it. But doing a boring, repetitive exercise with the sole intent of increasing your heart rate for an extended period of time may not be much fun. As a result, many people begin a cardiovascular exercise program and quite quickly abandon the effort. Once again, sustainability may be the most important part of any exercise program. If you won't continue doing it, then the program is of limited value.

There are, however, many other health benefits that could be realized from an exercise program.

If you engage in strength training, then you will be applying some type of load to your muscles, joints, and connective tissues. This can make you stronger and more resistant to injury. This is assuming that you don't overdo it and tear, strain, or injure the tissue. Injury and associated pain might make you stop training. Once again, if your exercise program is derailed due to injury, then will you be able to get back on the horse and resume your training? Consistency is required of your program if you are to be successful. How much load should you apply to your movements in order to get the health benefits of increased strength? Choose the amount that will take you out of the comfort zone and into the learning zone. In other words, the amount of weight should be whatever it takes to cause improvement. Look at the weight as you would a drug. Too little will not help, and too much will be bad for you.

Mobility training will also do wonders to improve your overall health and well-being. Group activities such as Tae Kwon Do or team sports will challenge your ability to move and react. These types of activities will also invariably challenge your cardiovascular system. You might find such an activity to be fun.

How do you know if your exercise program or training activity is good for you? The answer is whatever makes you better will make everything better. Perform some kind of self-assessment prior to your activity, and repeat the assessment after your activity. If your range of motion, strength, balance, or vision improves, then the activity was good for you. If your abilities decline, then the training was not good for you, and you did not become a better athlete. You should feel better and move better as the result of your training.

Mental Challenge

Our brains control our movements. Challenging our minds with complex movement patterns will help keep them sharp. The sensory inputs from our bodies — proprioceptive, visual, and vestibular — are all very active, and the brain is processing the associated data as we move about. The brain follows the same use-it-or-lose-it rule as our muscles, bones, and connective tissues. Therefore, one goal of our exercise program might be to purposely provide this type of stimulus to our central nervous system. Moving our bodies in complex ways will help us maintain or improve our three-dimensional awareness of our bodies in space. This ability will allow us to engage in whatever type of play we desire and will enable us to learn new sports skills more readily.

The cerebellum is a small structure located at the base of the skull that accounts for about 10 percent of the brain's total volume. However, there are more neurons in the cerebellum than in the rest of the brain. This means that the cerebellum is a very important structure. The cerebellum is responsible for timing, coordination, and refinement of motor skills. Recent research indicates that the cerebellum provides similar function for other brain activities, such as speech, memory, and visualization.[39] According to the *New England Journal of Medicine*, brain-stimulating leisure activities can reduce the onset of Alzheimer's disease and dementia.[40] In other words, it is possible that complex physical exercise such as ballroom dancing could improve the function of the cerebellum. This in turn can make the rest of the brain function better. One of the things you might want to get out of your exercise program is sensory stimulation and mental challenge.

Social Interaction

Humans are social creatures. We seek out the company of like-minded individuals. Exercise can be a social activity wherein we tap into the energy of those around us. This is the underlying basis for team sports and other group exercise activities. We feel better about ourselves when we receive tacit confirmation that what we are doing is cool, trendy, and acceptable. We may also push ourselves to achieve new levels of skill, fitness, and physical abilities in order to win. Humans are generally competitive. If someone else can do it, then we might think we should be able to do it too.

Another interesting thing often happens in these group training environments — we have fun. Tapping into the enthusiasm of others creates an enjoyable experience, and we seek to repeat this time and again. It is therefore more sustainable.

---

[39] "Harvard Research Shows How the Cerebellum Regulates Thoughts," Christopher Bergland, *Psychology Today*, May 21, 2016, https://www.psychologytoday.com/blog/the-athletes-way/201605/harvard-research-shows-how-the-cerebellum-regulates-thoughts.

[40] Verghese et al., "Leisure Activities and the Risk of Dementia in the Elderly."

Some people seek out a particular type of exercise simply because of the type of people they hope to meet there. We might want to look good so that we can find a date. So too we might want to go to a yoga studio, ride a bicycle in the MS-150, join a bowling league, or put on a Tae Kwon Do uniform so we can find date. Our desire for social interaction can be a significant motivation for our exercise program.

Mobility and Balance

One of the goals of this book has been to introduce the concept that all our joints, muscles, and bones exist for a single reason—movement. To keep the brain happy and, in fact, to be healthy, we must be able to move all joints through their designed ranges of motion. One of the reasons we have hands, arms, feet, and legs is for the purpose of moving our bodies. Push-ups, pull-ups, squats, and the like, all move our bodies through space as a result of force applied through our limbs. This is the essence of mobility.

You can be very strong and have lots of endurance but not be mobile. Likewise, being lean does not ensure mobility. If you want to be mobile, then your exercise program must include activities that challenge all your muscles and joints and move your body in a wide variety of ways. Mobility training should be a high priority in your exercise program if you want to become a better athlete and improve your health and well-being.

Balance is an integration of our movement skills together with the processing of sensory inputs from the proprioceptive, visual, and vestibular systems. I mentioned Scott McCredie's book, *Balance*, in chapter 2. This is an excellent introduction to how the brain and the body work together to create a sense of balance. Good balance allows us to move like an athlete—fearless and confident. Compromised balance forces us to move slowly and with a constant fear of falling.

Our exercise program must stimulate our vestibular system. This means we must turn around, lean back, lie down, roll over, and so forth. If we never turn our heads (or our bodies), then we will learn to be afraid of doing this. We will easily become dizzy. When we were children, we loved to spend time on a swing. Why? This stimulates the vestibular system. For the same reason, children love to turn around in circles until the world is spinning, and they fall down on the ground with laughter.

Whenever we are turning or getting up and down, we also experience a lot of visual stimulation. Our eyes and the information they are processing are supposed to provide us with accurate information about the world in motion. Does your training program stimulate your visual senses, or are you mostly sitting, lying, or standing in one place while you exercise?

Dancing and martial arts both provide high levels of visual and vestibular stimulation. In fact, I often think of martial arts practice as aggressive dancing. Similar benefits can be obtained from skating, gymnastics, and a variety of team sports activities. The essential skills we must practice are turning around and focusing our vision on objects.

Counteractives

Counteractives is a term I have coined to mean exercises we should do to counteract the adverse adaptive changes of our lives' activities. Whatever you are doing all day will be causing your body to adapt. Some of this adaptation may not be good for you.

Take as an extreme example someone who practices the bench press with heavy weights every day. This is a pushing motion performed in a lying position. This athlete may develop very strong wrists, arms, shoulders, and pectoral muscles. But for a healthy balance and symmetry, the athlete should perform pulling motions as well so that the muscles on the back are developed equally.

For most people in today's modern world, you will see a commonly occurring set of adaptions that are unhealthy. These adverse adaptations are the result of too much time spent sitting at a computer and from wearing overly restrictive, supportive, and cushioned shoes. Here are some things I see in client after client.

1. The chest is collapsed from spending time hunched over a computer. This causes the middle back, or thoracic spine, to be rounded forward. Breathing will be compromised by the time spent in this position.

2. The shoulders are moved forward, and the arms are internally rotated. This is encouraged by reaching for our keyboards and the mouse and by the arms on our chairs.

3. The hips are flexed in the seated position and will not fully straighten when the athlete stands up. Part of this is because our glutes are turned off while we are seated, and we no longer have the ability to turn them on when we stand up.

4. The feet are usually something like clubs on the ends of our legs. The feet are supposed to be strong and mobile and to absorb the shock incurred when we walk or run. But years spent with our feet tightly bound up in restrictive shoes has robbed us of this most-important ability.

5. The head and neck are moved forward while in the seated, computer-gazing position, and they remain that way when we stand. We are designed to stand erect with our head over our shoulders. In this

way, we can move better and react more readily to threats from our environment.

There are more of these adverse adaptive changes caused by the office-centric lifestyles we lead. However, you get the idea. One of the most important things that your exercise or training program can do to make you better and healthier is to help undo the adaptations described in this list. Performing counteractives, or exercises specifically designed to reverse this unhealthy adaptation, will greatly improve your athleticism and well-being. Instead of evolving into a creature whose only abilities are to send texts or e-mails and to type on a computer, you can maintain your quality erect posture, avoid chronic pain, and enjoy an active life.

Self-Assessment

One of the central premises of the Z-Health paradigm is that whatever makes us better makes us better. And, conversely, whatever makes us worse makes us worse. For example, if you have significant shoulder pain and you insist on doing push-ups, then here is what will most likely happen. You will "learn" that push-ups cause pain. You will become better at this skill of generating pain through the activity of push-ups. Furthermore, chronic pain *will not be ignored.* It is a creation of the brain to tell you to stop doing something or to do something differently. When you perform push-ups in pain, *there will be compensations.* You will not be performing push-ups with a quality movement skill but rather with some kind of work-around.

Therefore, the most important question you could ask yourself is "Is this exercise good for me?" Or "Does this practice make me better?" The answer to this question is so simple that it defies belief. All you must do is to listen to the nonverbal communication from your brain/body system. If it makes you better, then everything will be better — your vision, your balance, your strength, and your range of motion.

Time and time again, I have demonstrated this with clients. Here are a couple of examples.

Example 1. I have a client attempt to touch his toes. He observes how difficult the effort is and how far he succeeds in reaching. Then we perform some foot mobility drills. This is completely unrelated to the toe-touching activity, right? Then I ask the client to touch his toes. Voila! His forward bend improves.

Example 2. I have a client hold his arms out to the side and slowly move them forward. He observes how far the arms must move forward before he can see his hands with his peripheral vision. Then we perform some breathing drills that will improve the way he uses his diaphragm. Then I ask the client to perform the peripheral vision test again. Very often, the peripheral vision will improve, even though breathing seems completely unrelated to the client's vision.

I am sure you get the idea. One push-up, pull-up, or squat may make you better. Ten of them may make you worse. How many should you do? The answer is that it is up to you, and it depends on your training goals. But here is what is most important: your training session should make you better. If you leave your practice session in pain, hunched over, and moving poorly, then you will spend hours or even days adapting to your new, poor movement skills.

Now, I am not telling you that you should not push yourself. I am a big fan of mental toughness. I simply want to help you achieve results and to become the incredible athlete you were destined to be. If you break yourself day after day and workout after workout, then you will most likely end up as a broken former athlete. I believe that each of us has an infinite capacity for workload and quality movement skills — in other words, each of us can be exceptional athletes. But this requires the application of intellect and wisdom to our training. Push sometimes. Rest often. Get better every day.

Paradigm Shift

The first forty years of my training were conducted under the basic premise of "no pain, no gain." This meant two things. First, if you were not experiencing significant discomfort, then you simply were not training hard enough. Muscles were supposed to be sore or cramping, and your lungs must be burning. Second, if you were bruised, sore, had pulled muscles, or other injuries, then you must ignore the pain associated with these ailments.

Years of training with this overriding viewpoint made me really good at ignoring or misinterpreting the pain I experienced. Often, things that should have been really painful made me laugh because they tickled.

I now know that pain is an action signal created by the brain. The discomfort that we can experience as a result of our athletic activities falls into several distinct categories. Each of these types of discomforts requires a unique response appropriate to the meaning or cause of the pain experience. Here are some of the different pain events or uncomfortable experiences.

1. Discomfort associated with intense or extended muscle usage (including muscle cramps).

2. Shortness of breath resulting from heavy exertion.

3. Muscle soreness resulting from previous hard training.

4. Pain associated with tissue damage, such as pulled muscles, torn ligaments, cuts, and bruises.

5. Uncomfortable feeling associated with stretching activities.

6. Chronic pain.

I am a strong proponent of developing mental toughness in athletes. Kim Budzik, a friend and client whom I respect greatly, annually competes in the Badwater Ultramarathon. This 135-mile foot race of insanity starts in the desert of Death Valley and goes up and down mountains. Temperatures of more than 120 degrees Fahrenheit are common. Winning times range from twenty-two hours to thirty-three hours, and there is a forty-eight-hour cutoff time. Judging from these race details, I expect she might experience a few discomforts such as dehydration, blisters, pain, vomiting, stress fractures, overheating, and sleep deprivation. Am I recommending this? No. But I am proud to know someone who pushes herself to these extreme levels in order to excel. To be successful in any competition requires the elite athlete to possess a strong spirit. However, ignoring discomfort or pain can cause an undesirable outcome.

Unacknowledged pain represents a risk/reward decision. Do this at your own risk.

Notice that not all discomfort represents gloom and doom. Stretching, for example, can be quite uncomfortable, but the risk is usually low, assuming you are not pushing too hard or too far. As soon as you stop the stretching activity, the discomfort magically disappears. Of course, if you were to stretch too hard or too fast, then you could pull a muscle, damage a tendon or ligament, or tear something inside a joint. But this is quite a rare event.

Chapter 10: The Unique Z-Health System

There are many movement-based systems currently being promoted in the United States and around the world. What is so special about the Z-Health system? Simply put: Z-Health is the only brain-based training system.

The first thing implied by the previous statements is that other systems are focused on an output. The brain is in charge of everything, and movement is one of the outputs of the central nervous system. It is creating complex movement scenarios and then sending electrical impulses out to your muscles so that you can enact the desired motion. A Z-Health trainer will certainly be aware of your movement patterns and will work to help you improve those, but the primary focus of a Z-Health trainer is the inputs. The quality of the information that comes into your brain will have a direct bearing on the quality of your movement skills — just one of the brain's outputs.

One of the things that your Z-Health trainer will frequently employ to help improve your athletic performance or reduce your chronic pain experience will very likely be some apparently simple joint mobility techniques. All movement causes sensory input to be generated from your skin, fascia, joints, balance system, and vision system. The point of these exercises will be to provide specific, high-quality inputs to your brain and central nervous system. These new stimuli will cause a change in the way the brain understands your brain/body system and its ability to perform. Changes to performance, movement quality, or perceived pain can be realized almost instantaneously.

Since Z-Health trainers are focused on sensory inputs to the brain and the central nervous system, they may utilize a variety of other systems in order to find ways to make rapid changes. These other sensory input systems include the visual system, the vestibular system (or inner ear or balance system), the respiratory system, and the peripheral nervous system throughout your joints and fascia.

Three of the most amazing and unique tools that a Z-Health trainer will employ in his or her brain-based methodology are:

- threat reduction (or modulation);
- threat inoculation; and
- reassessment.

Let's take a look at these three instruments and how they can be used to improve your athletic performance or reduce chronic pain.

Threat Reduction

In chapter 7, you were introduced to the concept of the learning zone. This is the idea (represented by concentric circles) that there are three modes in which we can operate: the comfort zone, the learning zone, and the panic/danger zone. When we are in the comfort zone, there is insufficient novelty, stimulus, and challenge, and we do not grow, learn, or improve. By contrast, the panic/danger zone is a mode wherein we are under too much threat, and our fight-or-flight response takes over. In this state, our system reacts reflexively to ensure our survival. This may mean feeling panicked, having excessive tension, producing "bad" hormones, or exhibiting a lack of mental focus. The point of the learning zone concept is that we are best able to "learn," improve our skills, or grow new neural connections when we are between these two extremes.

Most people are not getting the most out of their training because they are constantly operating in the panic/danger zone. There are simply too many threats to the brain and the central nervous system, and we must constantly deal with these. We are unable to make improvements in ourselves because we live in survival mode. You are undoubtedly aware of some of these threats: stress and pressure from your job, tension in your relationships, and pollutants in the atmosphere. But another extremely important source of threat to the brain/body system is your sensory inputs. If you cannot move well, your balance is compromised, or your visual system is suboptimal, then your brain will correctly determine that your survival is in jeopardy. All your sensory input systems must be functioning well in order for you to be healthy and athletic.

Z-Health trainers will provide you with specific, sensory-targeted drills that will reduce the threat to the central nervous system. When this happens, it is like taking the brakes off your high-revving Ferrari. You will perform better. You will move from the danger/panic zone into the learning zone. You will begin to improve.

Threat Inoculation
The goal is to remove all threats and stress, right? No, that is not the objective.

Our goal is to improve the system, to reduce or eliminate pain, and to become more athletic. This means to be stronger, have better balance, increase our range of motion, and gain stamina. We will be healthier if we are more resilient.

But to improve our abilities and to reduce our chronic pain experiences, we must first reduce the unnecessary, unwanted, and extraneous threats to our system. We must improve the quality of our sensory inputs. These inputs include our visual system, our vestibular system, our respiratory system, and our peripheral nervous system. In other words, if we move better, more clearly, more accurately, and with more control, then there will be less threat to our central nervous system, and we will be more easily able to expand our tolerance to increased load (heavier weights), greater ranges of motion, and longer duration efforts. We will become more athletic.

Here is a simple example. Suppose you are performing push-ups with poor form. You want to become stronger and improve your endurance. To accomplish this, you are performing more and more push-ups each day. Practicing more poor-quality push-ups will simply increase the unwanted and unintentional stresses on your back, neck, shoulder joints, or hips. Your brain will complain more and more about the torture you are imposing on your body. However, when we improve the sensory input from these parts of our bodies, thereby improving the quality of our movements, we can now perform this drill without compromising the biomechanical system. We can increase the load, the range of motion, or the number of repetitions without damaging ourselves. In this way, we can improve our tolerance to this stress. We have successfully inoculated ourselves for this particular type of stress.

This is exactly what it means to become healthier and more athletic. If we improve, then we will be stronger, have better balance, and more endurance in whatever activity life throws our way. Here are some examples that are important to me.

- Suppose a friend asks me to help him move furniture. Can I carry heavy objects up and down several flights of stairs and load them into a moving van? Can I do this for eight or ten hours?

- If I have a major project at my job or a deadline that must be met, can I work eighteen or twenty hours in a single day and be productive for the entire time?

- If my children want me to chase them around the playground and climb on the monkey bars, can I keep up with them for several hours?

These are just a few examples of how being healthy and athletic can improve the quality of your life. Threat inoculation is one of the keys to improving our athleticism.

Reassessment

Why is the Z-Health methodology so successful? Because it is focused on the brain: both the inputs to the brain and the resulting outputs. If we provide proper and adequate stimulus to the central nervous system, then we will improve. We will get better. How do we know if the work or exercises we are doing are making us better? We determine this through the reassessment process. The Z-Health system is the *only* one that uses this particular element of evaluation to determine which efforts positively affect the brain, thereby ensuring that the drills we are doing help us perform better. This seems strange to me. The foundation of Western medicine is that medications are chosen based on a desired result and administered in the correct dosage for the patient's size, age, and condition. The patient is then observed to see if this desired outcome was achieved. If the patient didn't improve, then we must try a different treatment or adjust the dosage.

Exercise should also be thought of as a drug. We should first determine why we are doing it and what outcome we hope to achieve. Then we must evaluate (or reassess) to determine if it is working. Exercise can make you better or worse depending on which drill you do, how you do it, how much of it you do, and how often.

Your brain is evaluating your body's performance capabilities every moment of every day. What did you eat this morning? How well did you sleep last night? How long have you been hunched over in that chair reading this book? We simply cannot be assured that five sets of twenty push-ups are what we need to do *today* in order to improve. Perhaps today we need to do more. Or maybe we should cut back on our efforts and either try to improve the quality of the movement or simply take some time off for rest and recovery. Or perhaps we would be better served by working on something else entirely.

The Z-Health reassessment protocol is simply a way to ask the brain if it likes what we are doing. When we give our neurological control system what it needs and wants, it responds in a positive manner: we become stronger, our mobility improves, we have better balance, our vision improves, and more.

In order to gain insight into the central nervous system, Z-Health practitioners are trained to evaluate subtle details in the client's gait. Although walking seems to be a simple movement, it is quite complex and involves nearly every joint and muscle in the body. The way you walk will tell your Z-Health trainer much about your nervous system. Walking requires balance, awareness of our limbs, the ability to see what is around us, a process of integration within the brain, and much more. It is a full body/brain activity. But we generally don't think about how we walk. Our gait is largely performed automatically and outside conscious thought. The older, more primal areas of our brain control much of this movement pattern: the midbrain and the cerebellum. For these reasons, looking at the way our clients walk is a fast and simple way for us to determine if we have caused a positive change in the nervous system. Simply put: if the brain improves, then the client will walk better. The gait will be more efficient, more fluid, more balanced, and more athletic. Conversely, drills that are too much threat or cause pain will cause the quality of the client's gait to decline.

This is great news! Your Z-Health trainer will only give you drills or exercises that will make you better. Instead of a one-size-fits-all program of "do these exercises for this number of sets and reps because it made Bill look like Arnold," your program is about *you*. An exercise program is only valuable if it makes you better. If it breaks you, then it was not a good plan (even it if was good for Bill).

It is difficult, however, for you to evaluate your own gait because you cannot see yourself. Therefore, we need a different reassessment for you. When you are training on your own and you are performing any exercise, you might want to ask yourself, "Is performing this exercise or drill making me better?" After all, the point of every exercise program should be to make you better and to help you become healthier and more athletic. The reassessment protocol can be used even without a Z-Health trainer close at hand.

Any of the qualities we attribute to exceptional athleticism can be used for reassessment.

- Range of motion (or flexibility)
- Strength
- Endurance
- Balance
- Vision or perception skills
- Speed
- Mental acuity or memory recall
- Movement accuracy or quality

Of course, there is much more to exceptional athleticism, but you get the idea.

Here is an example of how you would apply the concept of self-reassessment during your solo training session. Suppose, for example, that you are training today on a pushing motion (such as a bench press, push-up, dip, kettlebell overhead press, or handstand press). How would you know if your training is helping you, and how would you know when you have gone too far with your efforts? Here are three options for you.

1. Before you begin your session, perform a couple of bodyweight squats. Simply observe the perceived rate of exertion (how hard it was), the balance you had during the movement, and the range of motion (or depth you achieved) during the squat. After you do a set of your planned exercises, repeat the self-reassessment. Evaluate the performance of your squat, and ask yourself, "Was it better, worse, or the same?" If your squat was better, then the brain likes the pushing activity, and it is improving the brain/body system. You are getting better. If your squat didn't change, then the central nervous system doesn't find this activity sufficiently stimulating or particularly novel. Unless you increase the load (weight or number of reps) or change the speed or the range of motion, you are probably not significantly improving your skill or abilities.

On the other hand, if your squat quality declines, then the brain is specifically telling you the following:

- You are using too much load (too much weight or too many reps).

- The work is requiring too great of a range of motion.

- The speed should be increased or decreased to help you improve your skill.

- There is too much visual or vestibular stimulation.

- You have a compromised respiration pattern.

Continued practice of an exercise or drill that is making your brain/body system perform more poorly is generally a bad idea.

2. Prior to the start of your session, bend forward and try to touch your toes or to put your hands on the floor. Then bend backward and reach as far back as possible. Note the difficulty, the balance, the speed, and the range of motion in both of these efforts. As before, perform your planned pushing exercises and then repeat the forward and backward bends. The question will be identical: "Was it better, worse, or the same?" When the answer is worse, continued training will be unlikely to help you achieve your goal of improvement.

3. When you first arrive at your training session, practice juggling some tennis balls. (This is my preferred self-reassessment method.) If you cannot yet juggle three balls, then just toss two balls from hand to hand. Juggling requires the central nervous system to integrate balance, visual perception, motor control, and sensations from the hands. It is also largely an automatic movement sequence, since you cannot "talk" yourself through the required motion. As in the other two options, make a note of the difficulty, balance, and feel of the effort. Alternatively, you can simply time how long you can juggle before you drop a ball. As before, start training, and periodically pause and retest your juggling skills. If the brain and the central nervous system like what you are doing, then your juggling performance will improve.

These are just simple examples. You can test your strength, balance, or range of motion in any way you choose. If you are doing push-ups, however, then the push-up drill itself will not be a good test. Eventually, you are going to become fatigued at that particular drill. Choose another, seemingly unrelated effort for your self-reassessment.

Whatever self-reassessment tool you choose to employ, it should be simple, not be too difficult, and not take a lot of time. If it doesn't have these qualities, then you are unlikely to do it.

It should be noted that pain is also an excellent tool for self-reassessment. For example, if moving your arm overhead causes you to feel pain, then you can use this movement as your assessment. How far can you move your arm before you feel pain? What is the level of the pain? If your pain experience declines, then the exercises you are doing are causing a positive adaptation to the brain/body system. Drills that are bad for you will reduce the range of motion or increase the discomfort.

The Neurological Action Loop

The Z-Health system is unique because it focuses on the structures of the brain; on inputs to the brain from the peripheral, visual, and vestibular systems; and on how the brain works to evaluate or interpret input and then generate outputs.

Why is this unique? A different system might focus on improving or changing your body's fascia in order to make you more mobile or to reduce your pain. Another system might focus on exercises performed with bands or weights to change muscle activation. Yet another system might emphasize releasing ligaments around the joints to try to realign those joints, thereby regaining or restoring their proper biomechanical function.

Any one of these approaches might work for you. And if they do, then that makes me very happy. Personally, I only want you to improve—to get better, stronger, healthier, and more athletic. Feel free to seek out qualified coaches who can help you with muscle activation, myofascial release, acupuncture, chiropractic, and the like. Anything that makes you better is a good thing. How can these varied approaches have success yet fail to be more universal successful? The reason is that they are not looking at the bigger picture. Other systems do not incorporate the *neurological action loop* into their way of thinking.

The neurological action loop works like this.

1. You move, you think, you feel, or you sense that something is happening in the world around you. These are *inputs*.

2. Based on your prior experiences, feelings, and memories, you determine the meaning and importance of the inputs you receive. This is the process of *evaluation* and decision making.

3. As a result of your brain's evaluation and decision-making process, you remember something, you act or move, or your brain creates a pain experience. These are *outputs*.

Once the brain creates an output, you feel pain, or you move — you once again find yourself at step one: you think, feel, or sense something. This is a feedback loop. You move. You feel. You evaluate. You move. And so on. The neurological action loop is the *input* causes *evaluation* causes *output* causes *input* loop.

Why is the neurological action loop important, and why is it so unique or novel? Because most systems want to address the biomechanical roadblocks to our performance. Many systems assure us that we have tissue that is not strong enough or not pliable enough to support our best athletic performance. This may, in fact, be true. But why do we have tissue like this? How did we develop it? How can we become better athletes? The answer is that our bodies adapt to the stimulus we receive from our movements in the world around us and from our brain's interpretation of what that stimulus meant. Until we actively and purposefully deal with our sensory inputs and the brain's processing of that information, we cannot expect to generate the highest quality outputs. We will be neither the healthiest people nor best athletes that we can be.

Chapter 11: The Z-Health Curriculum

I and many other Z-Health trainers have been able to help clients move better and to reduce or eliminate their chronic pain. To most clients, it seems like we are performing miracles or magic tricks. They are neither miracles nor magic tricks. And mostly, it isn't *us*. *We* usually don't actually do much more than provide instructions to clients. *They* do the work and perform the movements that make them better. This is an essential concept. Every individual is unique. What we do as Z-Health trainers is help the clients provide information to their own central nervous systems. Changes to the brain can occur very rapidly, in fact, almost instantaneously, and as a result, clients can often see magical changes to their strength or mobility. This can apply to chronic pain as well, and the pain often simply disappears.

Perhaps we can help the client retrain his or her brain, but ultimately it is up to the client. A music instructor can give you some shortcuts to learning how to play the piano. However, for this to work, you must want to play the piano, and you must diligently practice on your own.

The Z-Health Organization

Dr. Eric Cobb and Kathy Mauck started the Z-Health organization in 2003. It is an educational company with a goal of "creating health and fitness professionals in the top 1% of their respective fields." It does this by "providing individuals the framework and tools they need to optimize health and performance." In other words, the Z-Health organization provides information, training, and education. It is not, and this is an important distinction, a hospital or clinic where you can go to receive treatment.

The Z-Health organization offers many certification courses. However, this is all one integrated system. The information is simply broken down into manageable pieces so that the material will not overwhelm the student or client.

You can learn more about the history of the Z-Health organization and about Dr. Eric Cobb by reading his book, *The Fitness Professional's Guide to the NeuroRevolution*.[41]

---

[41] Eric Cobb, *Fitness Professional's Guide to the NeuroRevolution* (Tempe, AZ: Z-Health Performance Solutions, 2014).

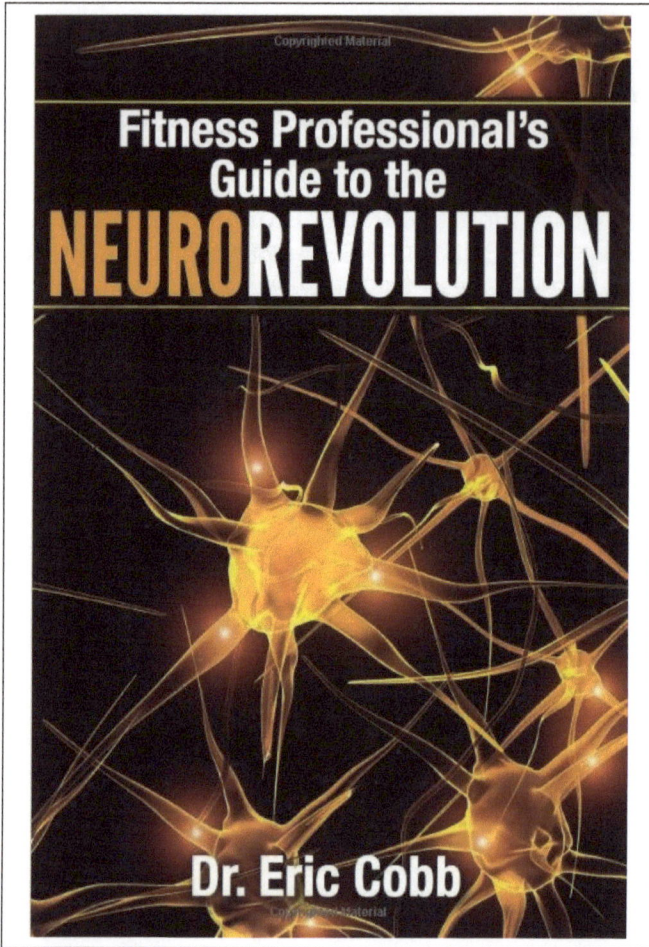

Fitness Professional's Guide to the NEUROREVOLUTION

Dr. Eric Cobb

The Basic Courses

The basic Z-Health curriculum consists of four course: R-Phase, I-Phase, S-Phase, and T-Phase. This section provides a brief introduction to some of the topics of these four certifications.

R-Phase is the *rehabilitation* course, and it introduces concepts like neuroplasticity and neural chunking and is primarily focused on reacquiring lost sensory input and motor skills on a joint-by-joint basis. Complex movements are broken down into their simplest components and then relearned in order to improve the quality of the movements.

I-Phase is the *integration* course. It introduces the vestibular system and advances the movement training to integrate the simple movements of R-Phase into more complex movements. As the movements become more complex, the client provides a much higher challenge to the central nervous system.

S-Phase stands for *sports*. In this course, the student is introduced to the concept of reverse engineering quality athletic movement. Sprinting and field sports are used as examples of how basic skills, required for exceptional performance, can be identified, broken down, and practiced in order to take athletes of any skill to the next level. During S-Phase, the extreme importance of the visual system is analyzed. We must be able to track a ball as it comes toward us. We must be able to process huge amounts of information from our visual field and to integrate it with our movement skills in order to perform well as an athlete. These skills can be practiced, and our visual ability can improve.

T-Phase stands for *threat*. In this course, the student is introduced to the concepts of threat assessment, threat reduction or modulation, and threat inoculation. The brain is in charge, and it is chiefly concerned with survival. This means that the central nervous system is constantly on the lookout for threats to the system. Threats to the system include allergens, job stress, poor movement skills, scar tissue from previous injuries, poor diet or nutrition, lack of sleep, and much more. When the system is exposed to too much stress, the sympathetic nervous system responds with the fight-or-flight reaction. This will almost always reduce our athletic performance. This course addresses shortcuts to find neurological inputs from the body that the brain perceives as threats.

Also covered in the T-Phase course is the topic of motivational interviewing. When you give a client an exercise or drill to do as homework and they do not do it, you will have failed as a coach. The manner in which we communicate with our clients is very important if we want to be successful as trainers. One of the key concepts of motivational interviewing is that our clients will listen to us much better if they feel heard. To do this, we must become better listeners. Another important concept is that what we say is less important than what the client hears. We must look for clues in what the clients say in order to determine what they heard. In Z-Health, the meaning of what we say is determined by the client's response.

An additional three-day overview course, "Essentials of Elite Performance," is also available. This is a sampler course that provides some of the materials from R-Phase, I-Phase, and S-Phase. This is an excellent opportunity to find out if the full Z-Health educational curriculum is something you want to pursue.

9S Specialty Courses

Z-Health introduces a rather novel concept: the client should not adapt to a one-size-fits-all exercise or training program, but rather, the program should provide exactly what the client needs in order to maximize his or her improvement. This puts the athlete at the center of the training plan. The 9S Athletic Development Model says that there are nine important aspects that influence an athlete and affect his or her progress.

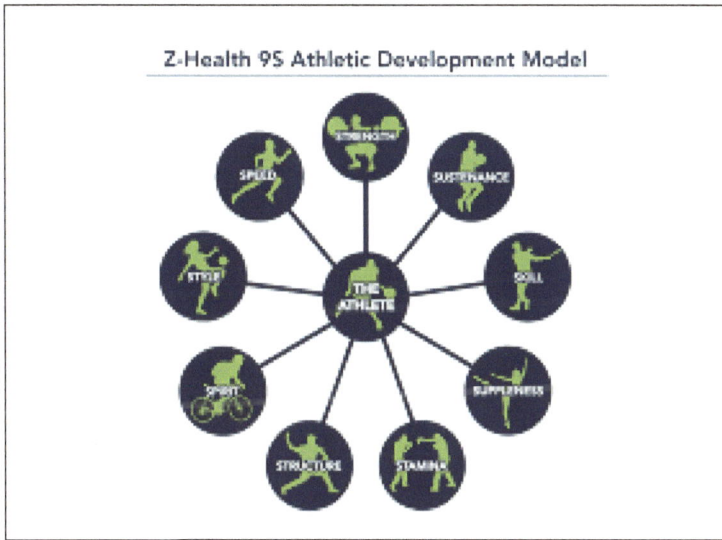

Z-Health 9S Athletic Development Model

The choice of what the athlete works on should be determined by the desired goals and by which training element will provide the best results. The nine elements of the 9S system are:

- strength;

- suppleness;

- sustenance;

- spirit;

- speed;

- skill;

- style;

- stamina; and

- structure.

The concept here is that the athlete is at the center of the 9S universe. And the needs of the athlete determine which one of the 9Ss we look to in order to improve the performance and health of the athlete. Why work on the athlete's strength if what the athlete needs is more stamina? Why spend time on stamina if the diet, or sustenance, is poor? Visualize a circle with a photo of your client in it. Surround this athlete's circle with nine more circles, each one representing one of the 9S elements. Now, look for weaknesses in the athlete, determine which of the 9S elements will improve the client, and work on that skill or function.

This is difficult. Most of us prefer to work on those things that we are already working on. We are comfortable with this approach. Most of us prefer to work on our strengths. If I am good at push-ups, then I really enjoy practicing push-ups. This builds my self-confidence by reinforcing the concept that I am good at push-ups. I am proud of myself. Others around me can clearly see that I am good at push-ups and may compliment me on my ability. But what if practicing push-ups is not the best way to use my time and energy? Perhaps practicing push-ups actually makes me worse at tennis, golf, or cycling. We must check our ego at the door and identify our objectives. If what we want to do is to get better, then we must do those things that will make us better and not those things that feed our ego.

In order to reduce the number of courses, the 9S certifications are often combined into two of the elements. What follows are the current 9S course offerings.

Strength and Suppleness
Are strength and flexibility mutually exclusive? Certainly not. In fact, the two concepts are closely related. Often, the thing that is keeping us from being stronger is the lack of flexibility or suppleness. Similarly, our lack of flexibility is not the product of our muscles being too short. Instead, we may have excessive tension in the opposing muscle groups.

In the strength section of this certification, you will learn how the brain is responsible for the amount of exertion or contractile force that a muscle group can produce. This is based on such variables as repeated training, day-to-day variations in health and stress levels, and sensory inputs from many areas of the body. For example, Golgi tendon organs are located at the area where muscles connect to or change into tendons. The Golgi tendon organs sense the amount of stress applied to the tendon via muscular contraction. The response to the intense contraction and its subsequent detection by the Golgi tendon organs can be to reduce the available contraction of the muscle group. In other words, if the Golgi tendon organs are activated, then you may not be able to strongly contract or increase the contraction of the associated muscle group.

Another of the many interesting concepts introduced in the strength section is that of occlusion therapy or occlusion training. This methodology involves training a muscle group while external devices, similar to a tourniquet, are purposefully employed to restrict the blood flow to the area. Exercises performed under the proper protocols encourage muscle hypertrophy. Larger muscles are exactly what bodybuilders want. The reason for this phenomenon appears to be that intense exercise and heavy loads require that the muscles contract strongly under a similar condition of insufficient blood flow. Therefore, purposefully restricting the blood flood allows exercises of even lower loads or intensities to encourage the same response of muscle growth.

If you are interested in improving your flexibility, then a wide variety of protocols for increasing your range of motion are explored in this certification. Some training activities are very effective but quite intense, while others cause less discomfort but require more extended effort in order to achieve significant improvement. As with all physical skills, the brain is the primary controller for your flexibility. When you are completely relaxed, your muscles are quite pliable and have a greater range of motion. What prevents you from being flexible? Usually, it is excess and unnecessary tension. Where does this tension come from? It is an automatic response from your brain to ensure your safety. Therefore, if we can convince our brain that it is safe, then it will allow us to move into a new (and possibly extreme) range of motion.

Recall the example of the straddle splits I was able to achieve as described in chapter 3. A bit of new sensory information made a world of difference. This new information, sent to the brain, said that it was safe for me to increase my range of motion. Please note that I was already close to the splits prior to this effort. But an increased range of motion is usually a combination of increased contraction of the active muscle group coupled with greater relaxation of the antagonistic muscle group. The brain controls both of these abilities, and it does so based on information from our sensory inputs and prior experience.

Sustenance and Spirit

Sustenance is the topic of how food and nutrition affect us and how it can enhance or impede our performance. Much of the information we hear and see via mainstream media and commercials is designed to sell us products. Diets, and how many carbohydrates, proteins, and fats we should consume, are discussed. You will also look at supplements and vitamins and how they affect the processes inside your body.

The topic of spirit is included with sustenance because they are closely intertwined. Most of us know that we will not lose weight and be the lean beach machine we want to be if we eat cheesecake every day. However, telling a client not to eat cheesecake does not help the client stop eating cheesecake any more than telling a smoker that smoking is bad for him or her. What do we need? Spirit covers the concepts of behavioral change and looks again, in depth, at motivational interviewing techniques. The idea of change must come from the client, and how we present ideas to him or her directly affects the likelihood that changes can begin. One of the great opportunities this certification provides is time to practice this skill with other humans. You will no doubt be surprised to discover that, even when you know they are being used on you, these techniques are highly effective. You will, in fact, learn to use these techniques on yourself to help you achieve new, positive changes in your life.

Speed

How do athletes improve their reaction time and speed? These are some of the questions addressed in the speed course. Speed is not only about sprinting but also includes the fast muscle contractions required for tennis, baseball, and boxing.

One of the factors that limits our reaction speed is our visual skill. The ability to rapidly track objects or people through space and then clearly focus on them can improve or limit our response. You will learn drills and be introduced to equipment that can be used to enhance your speed training efforts.

Skill and Style

Skill and Style addresses the differences among athletes and emphasizes their variations as they approach their chosen sports. Learn how to reduce the orientation time and to help your clients become proficient at any sport.

Introduced in this course is the OODA (Observe-Orient-Decide-Act) loop developed by US Air Force Colonel John Boyd. By using these techniques, you can seemingly know what your opponent is going to do before he or she does it.

Learning new skills can be fun, interesting, and exciting, but wouldn't it be great if you could significantly reduce the amount of time required to become proficient? That is what this course is about.

Stamina

Stamina approaches the subject of how endurance athletes can improve their ability to manage energy stores over the long haul.

What allows us to endure? What system fatigues and fails first? We need to identify the weak link in our system and to improve the stamina of that part of our athletic performance. These areas include:

- muscular stamina;

- cardiovascular performance;

- visual endurance;

- the ability of the central nervous system to resist fatigue; and

- how respiration affects our ability to continue our effort.

Respiration is essential for our ability to endure. When we breathe, we bring oxygen into our bodies, and this is essential for our ability to convert our stored chemicals into energy. Our breathing also expels large amounts of the by-products of our exertion: carbon dioxide. Carbon dioxide does two important things. First, it is the driver that tells us we need to breathe. You may have thought a lack of oxygen would make you breathe more, but this is untrue. If you replace all the oxygen in the room with nitrogen, then you would breathe quite normally while you died from lack of oxygen. However, when the atmosphere becomes rich with carbon dioxide, you will begin to pant. Second, carbon dioxide levels in your bloodstream affect the blood pH. An increase in carbon dioxide will cause your blood to become slightly more acidic. Your blood pH must be maintained within a very narrow range in order for you to survive. You can train your breathing, another movement skill, to better support your athletic endurance.

In addition to identifying and improving these areas, this course also examines the nutritional requirements of endurance athletes. Fine-tuning what your body needs in order to continue to perform over the long haul can be essential to success. Couldn't we all benefit from a little increased stamina? Maintaining focus throughout your difficult day requires stamina.

Structure

The structure course introduces the fascinating and complex topic of our brain's anatomy and how it functions. The course helps the student understand the different structures of the brain from the cerebrum to the cerebellum to the brainstem. Knowledge of these various structures and how sensory inputs are routed through the brain allows the Z-Health practitioner to make rapid positive changes to the athlete.

Z-Health is a brain-based system for improving athletic performance and reducing or eliminating chronic pain. Knowing how the brain works allows the Z-Health practitioner to use many shortcuts to cause rapid and dramatic changes. During this course, you will learn how to perform a fast yet comprehensive neurological examination to find areas of the brain that are functioning suboptimally. Using your new knowledge of the structure of the brain will allow you to stimulate the appropriate neural pathways to "wake up" those structures. The result: dramatic improvements in athletic performance.

The Master Trainer Program

There is an incredible amount of valuable material in the basic Z-Health program of R, I, S, and T courses. However, hearing and seeing the material is quite different from owning the material. The Master Trainer Program is a yearlong intensive course of study that leads to a mastery of the material in those courses. The Master Trainer Program culminates in the Live Training Week. During Live Training Week, the Candidate Master Trainer must demonstrate via oral questioning and practical demonstrations over a five-day period that he or she knows 90 percent of the material 100 percent of the time or 100 percent of the material 90 percent of the time. Oral exams are difficult and stressful; however, this process is necessary to ensure that the master trainer understands and can present the material under stressful conditions. The Z-Health Master Trainer Program, like all Z-Health educational programs, is constantly undergoing modifications to improve its effectiveness and to lead the fitness industry. Recently, a requirement for additional knowledge of gross anatomy has been added to ensure that master trainers have a requisite baseline of information needed for identification of structural issues.

This program requires commitment and dedication. At the conclusion of the program, assuming you pass, you will know the material, be able to apply it with your clients, and have a new paradigm or lens through which to view athletic training and personal improvement. And you will possess the confidence to apply your new knowledge to a wide variety of clients.

Evolution

One of the really good things about the Z-Health organization is that it is unafraid of change. New information is constantly being integrated into the course material. Courses are being restructured to make the presentation of the material more appealing, easier to learn, and more cost effective. As a result, the preceding information about the basic courses and the 9S specialty courses can and probably will change over time. Check out the Z-Health website at www.zhealth.net for the latest information on course offerings and content.

One of Dr. Cobb's visions has always been to create a community of practice, a group of like-minded individuals who will share case information and research in order to carry the Z-Health organization into the future while remaining on the cutting edge of applied neuroscience.

Why I Got Involved with Z-Health

I was training for an upcoming Tae Kwon Do tournament and was sparring with another black belt. I executed an instep kick toward my opponent's face, and — crunch — I heard and felt an unpleasant tearing in my left knee. I was certain I had torn some cartilage in the knee. I knew this because it wasn't my first time. So, I finished my training session. For the next several months, I taped and iced my knee and continued training.

Then I returned to the surgeon who had done two previous knee surgeries for me. Everything looked like a repeat of the previous repairs. They would put me under general anesthesia, perform an arthroscopic repair of the meniscus, and once again, I would be good to go.

I felt great when I woke up. I went home with a couple of crutches under my arms and began my rehab the next day. I was running within a couple of weeks. Then I noticed that things were not as I had hoped. Whenever I would start running, my knee hurt. It would stop hurting as I continued to run. However, when I finished running, there would be significant swelling. I returned to the surgeon and described my issues. He said that it might take another month to recover from the surgery. So I continued with my rehab exercises, my Tae Kwon Do training, and my running.

After four weeks, the symptoms were still the same. I returned to the surgeon and restated my complaint. He said to give it another six weeks. I thought this was a bit much, but I left the office with the intent to wait another six weeks. After all, he was the surgeon. He knew what he was doing. Didn't he?

After another six weeks—now about twelve weeks post-op—I went to see him again. It was at this point that he informed me why this operation was different from the previous ones. He said he had noticed some arthritis while he was in there, and he had decided to "polish the end of the femur." *What?* Isn't the smooth coating on the end of the bone supposed to be there? "It will grow back," he said. He then informed me that my knee was probably as good as it was going to get.

Over the next few years, my knee would swell whenever I did any significant physical activity, especially running. I was constantly icing it and wrapping it. I saw many more specialists to ask what could be done to restore proper function to my knee. They all said that I probably needed knee replacement surgery but that I was too active for this option. They recommended that I start taking it easy. Running and Tae Kwon Do were simply activities too strenuous for my knee. They didn't know why the surgeon "polished the femur," but they said that the knee was now a real mess, and there was nothing that could be done.

I was teaching at a three-day kettlebell workshop a few years later and coping with my condition by using a knee brace, ice, and anti-inflammatory medication. I had almost accepted that this was my new life. I was the guy with the bad knee that always hurt, had severely restricted flexion, and was constantly swollen. Of course, eliminating physical activity from my life was an unacceptable solution.

One of my students in the kettlebell workshop was a young woman named Katie. As I watched her training over the three grueling days, I was extremely impressed. This woman was one of the best athletes I had ever worked with. Katie was in excellent condition, very strong, and knew her body. She could learn new skills with ease. At the end of the workshop, we all went to a local bar for some adult beverages and a celebration. I had the opportunity to talk with Katie in a different setting. Sometime during the evening, I mentioned my knee issues. She reciprocated by telling me her story. She had fallen during a basketball game and seriously damaged her knee. She had torn both her ACL and MCL, the ligaments that stabilize the knee for lateral motion. She had undergone a couple of botched knee surgeries in an effort to repair the damage. Then she had an adverse reaction to the pain medication and developed an extreme pain syndrome. Her knee hurt even if someone was close to her knee. They didn't need to actually touch it.

I identified with her history and wondered how she coped with this situation. When I asked her how much pain she was in now, she answered, "None." I was shocked. This sounded a lot like my story. I asked her how she got out of pain, and she told me about Z-Health. She said that is why she had become a Z-Health master trainer. I asked her if she thought that Z-Health could help me. She said she was 100 percent certain that it could. A small ray of hope had been presented to me by one of the first Z-Health master trainers.

As soon as I could arrange it, I attended my first Z-Health workshop. Almost immediately, my pain began to subside, my swelling decreased, my range of motion increased, and I began to make more changes to my paradigm. Most of these changes are based on simple concepts. The Z-Health system is founded on cutting-edge neuroscience. Much of what has been discovered in the past ten years has not yet filtered its way through the educational system into mainstream medicine. But you don't need to understand all the science behind the system. Just use some of the concepts presented in this book to begin to change how you listen to your body, and as a result, change the way you exercise or train.

How a Z-Health Trainer Can Help You

Since the Z-Health organization in Tempe, Arizona, is not a hospital, clinic, or gym where you can go to get treatment, you might ask yourself how Z-Health can help you. Of course, I believe you should go through the educational curriculum offered by the Z-Health organization. This will help you understand the system and your body and might inspire you to take action to be the best, healthiest athlete you can be.

However, the Z-Health program requires dedication, and although it is certainly not inexpensive, the education is absolutely worth it. I was in the health and fitness business for nearly twenty years when I encountered the Z-Health program. I felt that I learned more in the first course, R-Phase, than I had in the previous ten years. I was astounded, overwhelmed, and amazed.

In the Z-Health system, years of study and research in strength, mobility and rehabilitation training, nutritional science, and an assortment of medical fields have been distilled and organized for you. During my college education, I felt that much of what I studied (and paid for) was not directly relevant to the degree I was pursuing. During your Z-Health education, everything you get during every course is directly applicable. And the material is current. The curriculum is constantly evolving to give you the newest cutting-edge science and information and how it can be practically applied.

Having said all that, you might not be interested or willing to invest the time, money, and energy to become a Z-Health trainer, but you might want to improve your athletic performance or to reduce or eliminate some chronic pain that you have been carrying around with you for years. In this case, you can and should seek out a Z-Health trainer.

Z-Health trainers are unique for many reasons.

1. Z-Health trainers know that the human body is amazingly adaptable. If you do the right thing, then you can expect incredible results. Some of these changes can happen instantaneously. Other changes, such as remodeling bone, can take years.

2. Z-Health trainers are willing and interested in hearing your story. Only by knowing how your journey brought you to this point can your trainer best assist you in making improvements. Our best source of information is you.

3. Z-Health trainers do not view the body as a collection of parts that can easily be repaired separately. Rather, the brain, the nervous system, the bones, the fascia, and the muscles comprise an integrated system. Vision and inner ear systems work with inputs from the entire body to allow you to move well through space.

4. Z-Health trainers are acutely aware that your occasional visit to them is less important than what you do all day, day after day. Ultimately, you are responsible for your own improvement. And that is a good thing. If you are waiting for someone else to fix you or to look after your well-being, then you are likely to be disappointed, or worse yet, misled.

What will a Z-Health trainer do for you? The goal will be to identify your goals and objectives, whether these are improved strength or performance, reduced pain, or something else, and then to look for whatever it takes to make you better. This is important to know at the outset. Whatever is holding you back from making progress may not be what you expect, and there may be (and likely are) many different things that will make you better.

The Path Forward

By now, throughout the pages of this book, you have been exposed to a lot of information that hopefully has begun to change your paradigm. Here are a few of the concepts we touched on.

Exercise should make you better. Certainly, this means you should move better. Perhaps it means you should be stronger, faster, more flexible, or have better balance. But exercise should make the mind/body system healthier. The goal of exercise is not to make you better at exercising. Although getting better at a particular exercise is not necessarily a bad thing. But what is exercise? How should you move? You should move every joint and every muscle in the body through every range of motion, every movement pattern, every speed, and under a variety of loads *frequently.*

Exercise or training can be used for threat inoculation. This means pushing ourselves to the limit so that we can expand the boundaries that limit us. Use self-assessment to determine if the challenges chosen during exercise are at the appropriate levels. We are looking for the sweet spot that will make us better. This will mean we are getting just the right amount of physical or mental challenge.

The brain is in charge. It is constantly processing information from your entire body. When the brain is happy with what you are doing—eating well, sleeping enough, and moving in a variety of ways—it will make you better, healthier, happier, and more athletic.

You must move. Movement is the key to life. Movement keeps all tissue pliable, keeps joints functioning, challenges the brain, updates the sensory and movement maps, and maintains the strength of the muscles and bones.

We must provide challenges to our vestibular system. This means we must change the orientation of the trunk: turn in circles, climb, get up and down off the ground, do handstands, and so on. This, hopefully, sounds a lot like play.

We must provide challenges to our visual system. Too much time is spent working on computers and iPhones with the eyes fixed at monitor distance or iPad distance. Play is an excellent way to get the visual system involved. Get outside and play catch, hide-and-seek, or some other sport that amuses, entertains, or challenges you.

Most people in today's society are subjected to too much stress, and these types of stress don't make us better. Stress reduction can improve our mental and physical skills.

There are two basic types of pain: acute and chronic. Acute pain is the result of an unhealed injury. Bleeding, bruising, or swelling is almost always associated with an injury. Chronic pain is different. It is the brain's way of communicating with you. Chronic pain is an action signal from the brain that says to do something or to do something differently.

The site of chronic pain may be unrelated to tissue damage or movement dysfunction. The level of chronic pain may be unrelated to the amount of tissue damage or movement dysfunction. In other words, when it comes to chronic pain, it is a pain experience created by the brain, and it cannot be trusted.

Our bones, muscles, connective tissues, and nervous system are constantly adapting to our efforts. Therefore, we must seek out those activities that will cause the desired adaptations.

The time you spend training and exercising must be used effectively in order to make you better. This means becoming smarter, more athletic, and healthier. You might also try to find ways to make your training more efficient so that you can spend less time in the gym and more time living life to the fullest. Changing your paradigm begins by questioning what you are currently doing. Are you getting better at exercise, or are you improving your brain/body system through the work you do each day?

You can change your paradigm and learn to see yourself and the world's athletes through the Z-Health lens. When you incorporate these concepts into your efforts, you can expect to feel better and to see rapid and long-lasting improvements in your health and athleticism.

Afterword

Check out these other principle-based books by Jay Armstrong also available from Amazon.

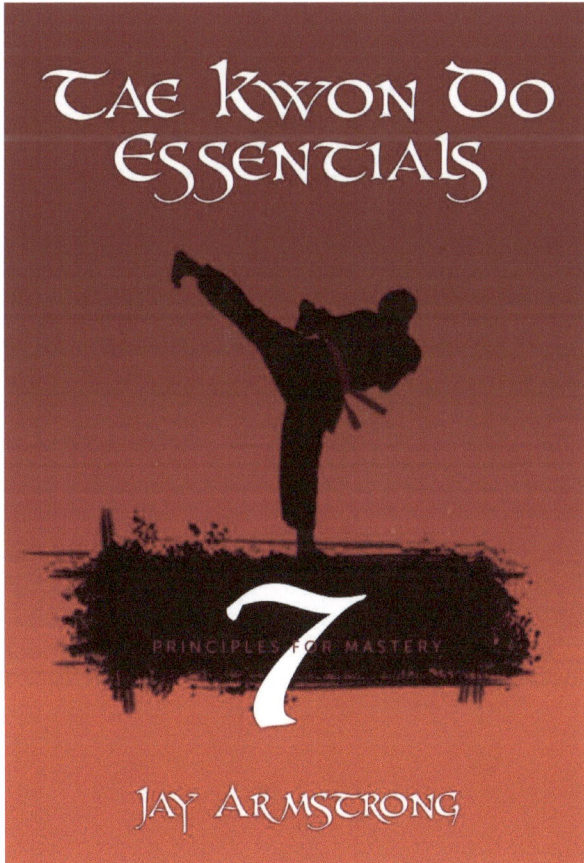

JAY ARMSTRONG

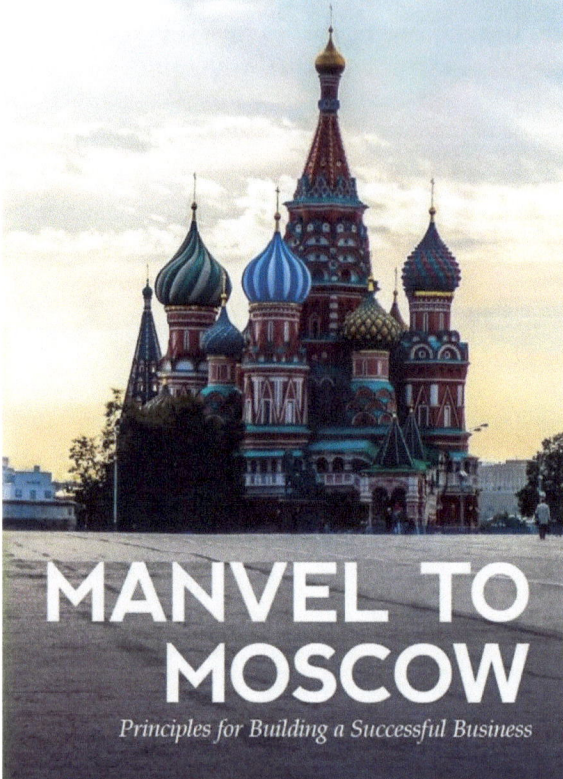

MANVEL TO MOSCOW

Principles for Building a Successful Business

Reviews

This is the book I wish I had read 10 years ago! It's my sincere hope that people read and apply the lessons in this book. Great job Jay!
  Max Shank – Master RKC Kettlebell Instructor, Owner Ambition Athletics

Jay provides an excellent description of what your body needs to function optimally. "What is Z-Health?" captures the essence of neuroplasticity.
  Dr. Stuart C. Hui - DC, ATC/L, Owner-Paradigm Performance Center

Great news! In "What is Z-Health?", Jay introduces corrective measures that anyone can use to undo the dysfunction caused by sitting in front of a computer, television or smart phone. I highly recommend that you read and apply this incredible wisdom!
  Dr. Bob Rakowski - DC, CCN, DACBN, DIBAK, Clinic Director of The Natural Medicine Center in Houston TX.

"What is Z-Health?" is an encyclopedia of neuroscience for lay people. This book is a primer for the future of the health and wellness fields. It has earned a special place in my reference library.
  MG Pogue, MA, ATC, ITAT - Athletic Trainer/Adjunct Faculty Ohlone College

This book is a treasure! It should be required reading for all coaches, personal trainers and athletes. Jay shares life-changing approaches to creating the you that you want to be.
   Lauren Brooks – Kettlebell Instructor, Owner of On the Edge Fitness

Jay delivers a deceptively simple yet profound analysis of applied neuroscience principles. He possesses the rare ability to boil down complex ideas into practical and effective tools that everyone can use. Reading this book will change your life.
   Nathan Baxter - 18-time Australian Powerlifting Champion and Elite Performance Coach

Ever wonder why your workouts do not bring expected results, why are you getting injured and why your injuries keep coming back, how could you be a better athlete or just a better version of yourself? Pick up a copy of "What is Z-Health?" Jay translates the science of neurology into simple language that can be applied to athletic training, performance and rehabilitation. It's a must read!
   Ildiko Varhelyi - RYT, PTA, LMT, Z-Health Master Trainer

www.ingramcontent.com/pod-product-compliance
Lightning Source LLC
Chambersburg PA
CBHW041220270326
41932CB00003B/5